Handbook of
Renal Investigations
in Children

Handbooks of Investigation in Children

This is a series of unique guides to the appropriate tests to be carried out in children with suspected disorders. Instructions for the performance and evaluation of tests are clearly explained. Each title is based on the authors' personal experience in the respective field and is devoted to the investigation of children only.

Careful reference to these titles in clinical practice will help both to eliminate inadequate testing and to ensure that the practitioner will obtain the maximum information from the investigations carried out. To amplify the explicit text, case histories or algorithms helpfully illustrate how the authors have used and interpreted investigations. These pocket-sized books are essential tools for all those involved in the diagnosis and management of childhood disorders.

Other titles

Handbook of Endocrine Investigations in Children
  I. A. Hughes
Handbook of Haematological Investigations in Children
  R. F. Stevens
Handbook of Neurological Investigations in Children
  J. B. P. Stephenson and M. D. King

Handbook of Renal Investigations in Children

C. M. Taylor MRCP, DCH
Consultant Paediatric Nephrologist
The Children's Hospital, Birmingham
Honorary Senior Clinical Lecturer
University of Birmingham

S. Chapman MRCP, FRCR
Consultant Paediatric Radiologist
The Children's Hospital, Birmingham
Honorary Senior Clinical Lecturer
University of Birmingham

WRIGHT
London   Boston   Singapore   Sydney   Toronto   Wellington

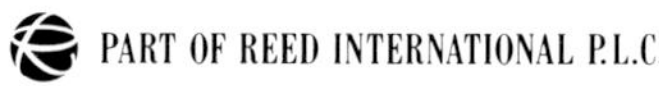 PART OF REED INTERNATIONAL P.L.C.

Wright
is an imprint of Butterworth Scientific

First published 1989

© **Butterworth & Co. (Publishers) Ltd, 1989**

British Library Cataloguing in Publication Data

Taylor, C. M.
 Handbook of renal investigations in
 children
 1. Children. Kidneys. Diseases
 I. Title II. Chapman, Stephen, *1953–*
 618.92'61

 ISBN 0–7236–0720–6

Library of Congress Cataloging in Publication Data

Taylor, C. M. (C. Mark)
 Handbook of renal investigations in children / C. M. Taylor, S. Chapman.
 p. cm.—(Handbook of investigations in children)
 Bibliography: p.
 Includes index.
 ISBN 0–7236–0720–6 :
 1. Pediatric nephrology—Handbooks, manuals, etc. 2. Kidneys—Diseases—Diagnosis—Handbooks, manuals, etc. I. Chapman, Stephen. II. Title. III. Series.
 RJ476.K5T38 1989   89–473
 618.92'61—dc19   CIP

Typeset by Latimer Trend & Company Ltd., Plymouth
Printed and bound in Great Britain by Butler & Tanner Ltd, Frome, Somerset

Foreword

We live in times of increasing clinical specialization, and of an accelerating increase in basic scientific knowledge on which these clinical developments are based. The urge to 'keep up to date' is present in all of us but, confronted every week in medical journals by new tests, new syndromes and the debunking of old precepts, it is easy to become defensive or even demoralized.

There is a need for experts in important fields to publish for the general reader up-to-date accounts of how to do it, and why. If these experts can write easily, and with the authority that comes from experience, then there should be a ready market for the product of their labours.

I believe that these criteria are met in full by the present publication. Drs Mark Taylor and Stephen Chapman investigate and treat children with renal problems every working day. They have developed a rational approach to the investigation of these children that is aimed above all at precision of diagnosis, but which seeks also to eliminate unnecessary investigation and discomfort. In the text the authors have also indicated clearly those investigations that should (indeed must) be available in all district general hospitals, and those which are best concentrated in tertiary referral centres.

The authors have told me that the book is aimed at the junior doctor in training. I can firmly assert that consultant paediatricians ought to read it as well.

Alexander S. McNeish
Leonard Parsons Professor of Paediatrics and Child Health,
Director of the Institute of Child Health,
University of Birmingham

Preface

The number of investigations available to help in the diagnosis of paediatric renal disease has grown markedly in the past decade, much of this growth being in the area of urinary tract imaging. Conversations with non-specialist colleagues and paediatricians in training indicate to us that this increase is often seen as complex or confusing, and supports our view that there needs to be a short text which puts renal investigation into a simple but up-to-date perspective. The good news is that most of the progress towards a definitive diagnosis in a renal patient can still be made from the history, relatively few physical signs and inexpensive elementary investigations. Much has been done recently to streamline renal investigations in childhood, and gone are the days of 24-hour urine collections and endogenous creatinine clearances.

We need no excuse for emphasizing the importance of a full history which will influence the speed and direction of further investigations. For example, the nephrotic child with an abrupt onset of oedema at 3 years of age has a 90% chance of having steroid-responsive minimal change nephrotic syndrome. By contrast an insidious onset in a teenager makes this diagnosis much less likely and demands closer scrutiny. Urinary tract infection ranges from an asymptomatic state through incontinence and micturition disturbance to the most prevalent renal-destructive disorder in childhood. Careful historical enquiry helps to determine how urgently to investigate and treat.

Two of the physical signs most relevant to renal disease are often passed over: the measurement of jugular venous and systemic arterial blood pressure. When presented with an oedematous, oliguric child the former assists in deciding whether this is a nephritic illness with an expanded vascular volume, or a nephrotic one with hypovolaemia. Immediate decisions about fluid management depend on this.

As far as the investigations themselves are concerned, the simple tests, when properly understood and applied, take the investigator very close to a definitive diagnosis. Too many children undergo invasive tests unnecessarily. An example is the child with persistent haematuria who is referred for cystoscopy when no attempt has been made to look for dysmorphic erythrocytes or casts in the urine, the presence of which clearly indicates a glomerular cause. Within referral centres for paediatric nephrology the dialogue between physician, urologist and radiologist has been the key to improving the diagnostic service for many children with nephro-urological disease. The advent of ultrasound, which is far more observer dependent than excretion urography, demands that the dialogue continues to grow not just in specialist but in all paediatric departments. The natural wish to use less invasive imaging techniques must be supported by a well-founded faith in the newer technologies. This will depend not only on their inherent strengths and weaknesses but also on the ease of access and the skill of the radiologist in performing and interpreting them.

This book, written for the non-specialist, gives the greatest detail to the simpler tests. Where special investigations are needed outline details are given to assist with the decision about referring to paediatric nephrological or urological services. The main part of the text is concerned with investigation techniques. The Appendices contain algorithms which we hope will put the tests themselves into a clinical framework. If readers have an inherent dislike of medical algorithms we can only apologize for this. In our view the alternative is to have case illustrations, and of the criticism that flow diagrams are too general and specific cases unrepresentative, we are more comfortable defending the former. In modern medicine any text has only a short shelf-life and the principles underlying a course of investigation will, we think, prove more durable than a single example frozen in time.

Acknowledgements

Our thanks must go to Kathleen Snow, Paul England and Jackie Harvey of the Department of Medical Illustration at Birmingham Children's Hospital and to Henry Buglass for the excellent work they have done in preparing the illustrations, tables and flowcharts. Mrs Veronica Penney typed much of the manuscript.

As always, our families were tolerant of the hours spent away from them and supporting when deadlines approached all too quickly. They deserve a special thank-you.

Contents

Abbreviations

ADH	antidiuretic hormone
AXR	plain abdominal X-ray
BSA	body surface area
BSP	bromosulphthalein
CMD	corticomedullary differentiation
CMG	cystometrogram
Cr	chromium
CT	computed tomography
CXR	plain chest X-ray
DMSA	dimercaptosuccinic acid
DTPA	diethylenetriamine pentacetic acid
ECF	extracellular fluid
EDTA	edetic acid
EMG	electromyography
EMU	early morning urine
ERPF	effective renal plasma flow
EU	excretion urography
FE	fractional excretion
GFR	glomerular filtration rate
HLA	human leucocyte antigen
I	iodine
ICRP	International Commission on Radiological Protection
LOCM	low osmolar contrast medium
MCUG	micturating cystourethrography
MIBG	meta-iodo-benzyl-guanidine
MSU	midstream urine
NRPB	National Radiological Protection Board
OIH	orthoiodohippurate
PJL	parenchymal junctional line
PRA	plasma renin activity
PUJ	pelvic-ureteric junction
RBC	red blood cell
RIA	radioimmunoassay
RNC	radionuclide cystography

ROI	region of interest
RPKD	recessive polycystic kidney disease
RTA	renal tubular acidosis
RVT	renal vein thrombosis
SPA	suprapubic urine aspiration
SRVR	segmental renin vein ratio
Tc	technetium
UIR	unit impulse response
US	ultrasonography
UTI	urinary tract infection
VMA	vanillyl mandelic acid
VUR	vesico-ureteric reflux
WBC	white blood cell
WKTT	whole kidney transit time

Chapter 1

Urine collection

Introduction

Appropriate examination of the urine remains one of the fastest routes towards the diagnosis of renal disease. In infants and young children the collection of urine samples presents obvious difficulties (Meadow, 1977). Children below the age of about 3 years are unable to void on demand at less than bladder capacity. Moreover all young children are readily intimidated by being asked to micturate in strange surroundings. For this reason it is important that children are investigated in the presence of a supportive parent and confident and relaxed nursing staff; compulsion is likely to be counterproductive.

Three factors influence the choice of urine collection method:

1. Age of the patient.
2. The requirement for microbiological investigation.
3. The urgency of investigation.

Bacterial invasion of the urinary tract is common. Up to 5% of females will develop a urinary tract infection (UTI) at some stage during childhood. The incidence in males is much less but it should be remembered that approximately 1% of all neonates develop UTI with slightly more males being affected than females.

The clinical expression of UTI in childhood ranges from an asymptomatic carrier state in which active renal disease does not occur, to an acute and severe inflammatory disorder of the renal parenchyma (acute pyelonephritis). Animal experiments indicate that in the latter prompt antibiotic treatment can allow recovery without parenchymal fibrosis, whereas delay is associated with the development of coarse renal scarring (Ransley and Risdon, 1981).

In clinical practice older children with the symptoms of acute pyelonephritis present early and are quickly treated. By contrast in children below 3 years of age signs of illness are less specific and there is the risk that the diagnosis is delayed. It is in this age-group, and in infants particularly, that renal scarring occurs. It follows that the diagnosis of UTI needs to be confirmed urgently in infants and young children in whom it is suspected (White, 1987).

At this age the disturbance of micturition which accompanies UTI is variable, some infants frequently dribbling small volumes of urine while others inhibit voiding for many hours at a time. A clean-catch midstream urine (MSU) sample is therefore more difficult to obtain, although it should be sought in all cases. In the sick infant in whom a clean catch is not immediately obtained suprapubic urine aspiration (SPA) should be performed. If the SPA fails to provide a sample one can repeat this after a short period in the hope that the bladder will by then contain more urine. On the whole this is preferable to urethral catheterization which can be a painful procedure in males, induce catheter shock and may contaminate the urine sample with urethral organisms. Antibiotic treatment must not be withheld pending urine culture results. This makes it more important that either a clean catch or SPA sample is obtained so that microbiological results will be unequivocal.

In other, afebrile infants in whom one is attempting to *exclude* a diagnosis of UTI a bag urine sample may suffice. Bear in mind the fact that 10% of bag urine samples when cultured give a false-positive indication of UTI and one must therefore be prepared to repeat the collection where there is doubt. It is inappropriate to rely on a single bag urine collection to identify positively UTI even if prompt microscopy of the specimen suggests the diagnosis. The algorithm on page 176 gives an overall scheme for urine collection in urinary tract infection.

The clean catch

In infants micturition occurs as a reflex stimulated by bladder fullness, and this can be provoked by sudden cold exposure. The well-prepared doctor or nurse will have a sterile universal container to hand when a baby is undressed for clinical examination or weighing. By this means a clean-catch urine sample may often be obtained. For neonates, another manoeuvre is to hold the child in ventral suspension and lightly stroke along the back parallel to the lumbar spine. If the child has a full bladder this may also provoke reflex voiding. In practice, however, the child will have been undressed by this time and one of the better opportunities for stimulated voiding will have just been missed. The fact that adhesive urine collection bags are widely available is no excuse for not attempting to get samples from babies by the above method. As will be seen below, urine bags have a number of disadvantages beyond their unpopularity with mothers.

Midstream urine collection

In older boys who are perhaps more used to voiding in public MSU collection presents few difficulties. Unless the patient has obvious balanitis there is no need to withdraw the prepuce or cleanse the glans. A sterile universal container is introduced into the urinary stream to collect the midstream sample. Older, cooperative girls are probably best to collect their own MSU so long as they are appropriately instructed. Unless the child has severe vulvitis or faecal contamination of the vulva there is no need for vulval washing. In neither sex should antiseptics be applied to the genitalia as these may contaminate the urinary stream and interfere with the culture of pathogens.

In younger girls it is easier to collect a midstream sample using a purpose-designed toilet in which the bowl is cut away at the back. During micturition the attending nurse can introduce a sterile foil gallipot mounted in a stiff wire loop ('fishing rod') into the stream without disturbing the child. For young potty-trained girls Huttunen, Mella and Makela (1970) developed an automated MSU collector. This resembles a normal child's potty but in the forward part of the bowl is fixed a ring into which a sterile foil gallipot can be placed. The child voids normally into the potty. The first part of the urinary stream runs directly downwards into the bowl, but as flow increases in midstream the trajectory is more anterior and reaches the sterile gallipot (Figure 1.1). For a time these automated MSU collectors were made commercially but many paediatricians and GPs have no doubt simply modified inexpensive children's potties.

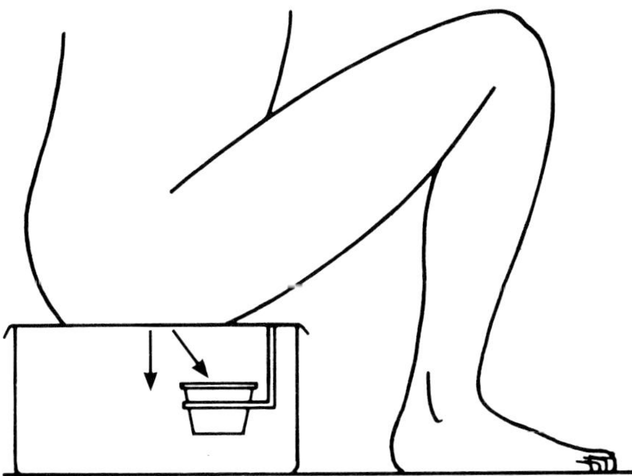

Figure 1.1 The automated MSU collector

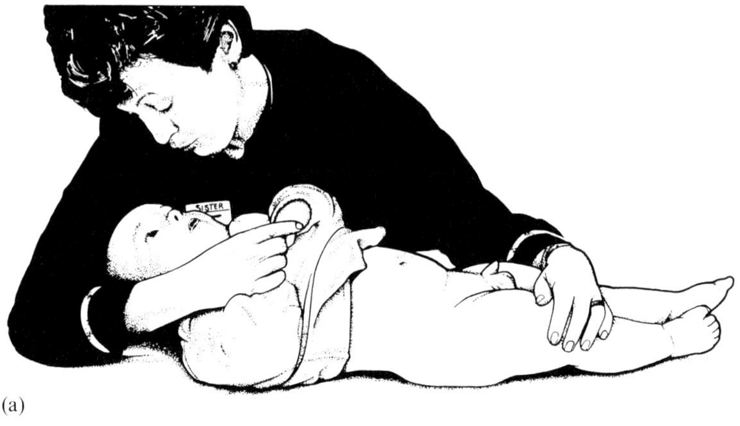

(a)

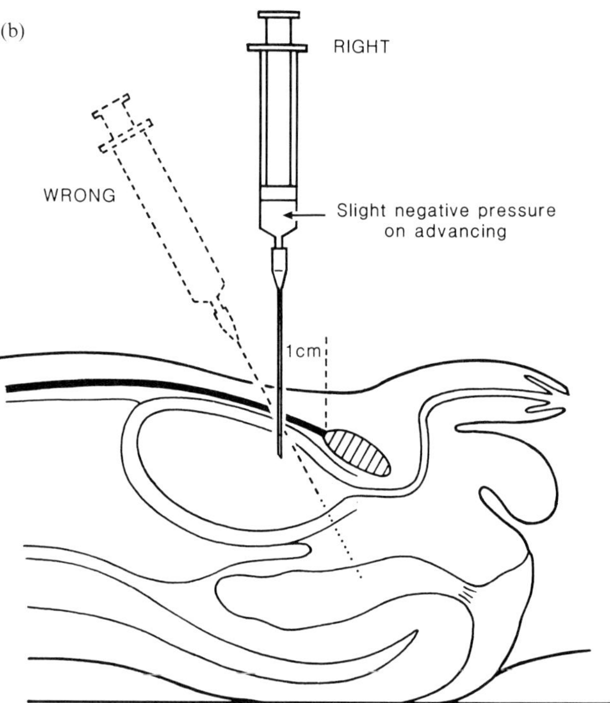

(b)

Figure 1.2 Suprapubic aspiration (a) Restraining older infants. (b) The procedure

Suprapubic aspiration

To perform an SPA satisfactorily it is essential that the child is held appropriately by the nurse to prevent movement. Whereas newborns are easy to immobilize, the older infant can be more awkward. In the preferred method the child lies supine on a firm surface such as an examination couch with the nurse sitting towards the head. One arm is placed round the child's shoulders and the nurse holds the child's hands across his or her chest thus preventing thoracic movement. With the other hand the nurse holds the child's knees together to prevent flexion at the hip. Thus restrained the infant has little opportunity to move pelvis or lumbar spine and the bladder therefore remains a stationary target (Figure 1.2).

The doctor positions the opened sterile universal container within easy reach in case the child voids prior to bladder puncture. The midline suprapubic skin is cleaned with alcohol and dried with cotton wool. Taking a 10-ml syringe with 21G needle the operator pierces the skin perpendicularly in the midline approximately 10 mm above the symphysis pubis. Once the eye of the needle is in the subcutaneous tissues the operator draws back gently on the syringe plunger to create slight negative pressure. Maintaining the negative pressure, syringe and needle are advanced perpendicularly. In this way the needle traverses the linea alba, avoiding the parietal peritoneum which reflects onto the dome of the bladder cephalad to the path of the needle, and penetrates detrusor muscle. As soon as urine wells up into the syringe the advance of the needle is stopped. Once an adequate volume of urine has been obtained, 1 ml is more than enough for microscopy and culture, syringe and needle are withdrawn.

Thus performed SPA is a safe procedure. Moreover, because the dome of the bladder contains no pain fibres it is no more uncomfortable than a venepuncture. There are two common errors that untrained operators encounter. The first is to angle the needle down towards the pelvis. The bladder is an abdominal organ in early childhood and any attempt to aim the needle caudally risks striking the trigone of the bladder, which may cause considerable pain. The second common mistake is to plunge the needle right through the bladder before creating any negative pressure in the syringe and then to aspirate urine on withdrawal. This has the potential for passing the needle into gut posteriorly and risks aspirating bowel contents along with the urine.

Bag urine collection

A variety of adhesive urine-collecting bags are currently available, one of the better known is the Hollister U-bag. This product is sterile and contains an inner envelope which acts as a one-way valve so that the voided urine falls to the base of the urine bag and cannot regain contact with the child's external genitalia. Urine is drained from the bag via a port covered by a tear-off seal. This also ensures that the sample is not further contaminated by the upper portion of the bag which has been in greater contact with the child's skin. In practice these theoretical advantages are very often lost because of inexpert use.

Before applying a urine bag the genitalia should be cleaned of any faecal contamination by washing with soap and water. The skin is then dried and the urine bag securely attached over the external genitalia making sure that the perianal region in girls is excluded. The adhesive collar is very sticky and it is a cruelty to apply these devices to broken skin; severe nappy rash is a contraindication to the use of these bags. The bag hangs between the child's thighs and should not be folded or crumpled. The infant is nursed, preferably in an erect position, by the parent. As soon as the child voids the bag is removed and the urine decanted into a sterile container.

A common error in the use of urine bags is to re-dress the child. This often means that the urine bag is not decanted quickly after the child has voided and in the meantime urine has become heavily contaminated by skin bacteria.

Catheter specimens

Instrumentation of the lower urinary tract carries the risk of introducing infection into the bladder, traumatizing the urethral mucosa and inducing catheter shock in which bacterial antigen gains access to the blood via the dense vasculature of the periurethral tissues.

The genitalia are cleaned with 0.5% aqueous chlorhexidine while the child is held in the lithotomy position. In females lubricant is not essential, but in males sterile 1% xylocaine or KY Jelly (Johnson) is helpful. Using strict aseptic technique a soft, fine feeding catheter such as a 5 French gauge Argyle is inserted into the urethral meatus and advanced until urine is seen to flow along it. In males pain is often experienced as the catheter turns in a cephalic direction on entering the membranous urethra. Involuntary tensing of the pelvic floor makes catheter advancement difficult; however, the application of gentle upward pressure over the perineum may facilitate bladder entry. Within a paediatric department it is good management for one or two of the experienced nurses to undertake all urethral catheterization, as by practising this skill regularly high standards can be maintained.

References

Huttunen, N. P., Mella, E. and Makela, P. (1970) Simple method for increasing reliability in diagnosis of urinary infection. *Lancet*, **ii**, 22

Meadow, R. (1977) Collecting urine for culture from children. *Journal of Maternal and Child Health*, **2**, 46–51

Ransley, P. G. and Risdon, R. A. (1981) Reflux nephropathy: effects of antimicrobial therapy on the evolution of the early pyelonephritic scar. *Kidney International*, **20**, 733–742

White, R. H. R. (1987) Management of urinary tract infection. *Archives of Disease in Childhood*, **62**, 421–427

Chapter 2

Urine microscopy and culture

Microscopy

Urine microscopy is a quick, reliable but under-used investigation. A simple microscope and counting chamber, if looked after carefully, will last a lifetime and, by saving unnecessary laboratory costs, the financial outlay for the microscope will be more than recovered. Every paediatric department, casualty or group health centre should have one and the medical staff, with minimal training, will confidently recognize urinary cells and organisms. It has been clearly shown that in the microscopy of fresh, uncentrifuged urine the appearance of leucocytes and bacteria together gives a good agreement with culture results (Robins *et al.*, 1975).

Figure 2.1(a) shows the measuring grid layout of a Fuchs–Rosenthal counting chamber. The half-silvered floor of the counting chamber is precision ground to a depth of 0.1 mm below the surface of the slide. When a glass cover slip is in place the volume contained between the grid lines is as shown. Using a small rod, or better a plain glass capillary tube as a pipette, freshly collected urine is introduced under the cover slip where it is drawn by capillary action to fill the counting chamber. If urine has been standing it should be shaken up to resuspend the cellular deposit, unless a specific search is being made for casts. Urates and phosphates may precipitate within urine, making microscopy difficult. The former can be cleared by rewarming the urine sample (hold the specimen under the hot tap for 2 or 3 minutes); the latter may be redissolved by adding a few drops of acetic acid.

With the × 10 objective lens, the larger cells can be identified confidently. *White blood cells* (WBCs) are recognized by their size and granular cytoplasm. *Squamous epithelial cells* are polygonal, larger in area than WBCs and have a distinct nucleus.

Casts tend to stick to the urine meniscus so that it is worth searching round the edge of the urine droplet for these cylindrical bodies. *Hyaline casts* made up of compacted proteins (principally Tamm–Horsfall protein) appear homogeneous compared with cellular

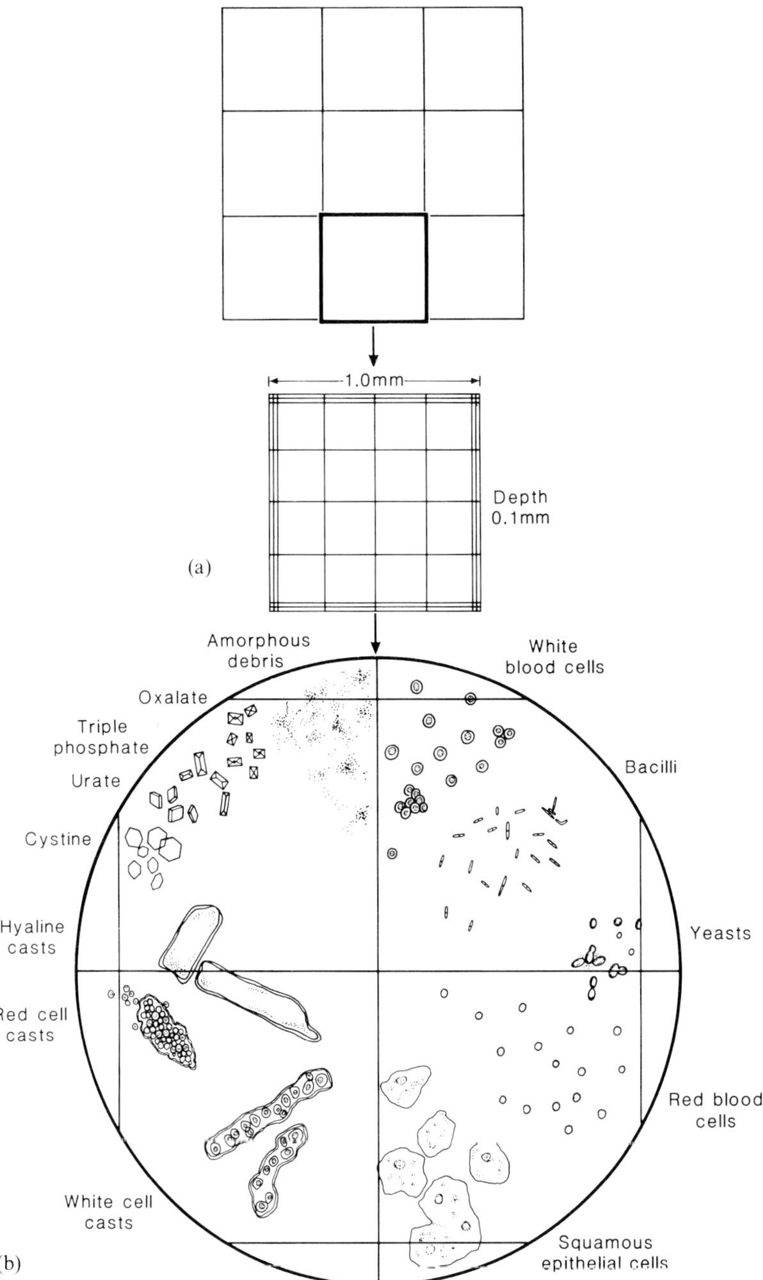

Figure 2.1 Urine microscopy. (a) Fuchs–Rosenthal counting chamber. (b) Microscopic findings

casts. However, the condensation of some proteins may give the cast a faintly granular appearance. Hyaline casts usually indicate a recent period of heavy proteinuria, but they are occasionally seen in normal individuals and in those who have become dehydrated. Sometimes hyaline casts are shed with adherent tubular epithelial cells on their surface, and in unstained preparations these can be mistaken for other types of cellular cast. They are a feature of acute tubular necrosis, interstitial nephritis or rapidly progressive glomerulonephritis.

With little experience *red and white cell casts* can be distinguished without resorting to staining, the WBC cast having a dense granular appearance compared to the red cell cast. They provide irrefutable evidence of renal bleeding and parenchymal inflammation respectively.

With the × 40 objective, *red blood cells* (RBCs) and microorganisms can be seen. It takes a few minutes for the RBCs to settle on the floor of the counting chamber. By focusing up and down one can be convinced by their biconcave shape. There is of course no nucleus and the cells are approximately two-thirds of the diameter of a WBC. In hypotonic urine RBCs may lyse leaving only their cell membranes (ghosts).

It is valuable to know if haematuria is glomerular in origin, and if red cell casts have not been found after a careful inspection of the urinary deposit, the appearance of the erythrocytes themselves may give a useful clue. Whereas red cells from the lower urinary tract have normal contours, those which have passed down the nephron are dysmorphic when viewed by phase contrast microscopy (Fairley and Birch, 1982; Rizzoni *et al.*, 1984). It is not a difficult matter for a clinician or laboratory staff member to become proficient at distinguishing between the two.

Microorganisms are best seen with the light source turned down so that they appear bright against a darker background. They tend to show Brownian movement but sometimes motile bacteria are seen. In urinary tract infection organisms are typically present in large numbers so that if a urine sample contained 10^6 organisms ml^{-1} one would expect to see an average of 25 in each small square in the counting chamber. Coliforms can be easily distinguished from chains of faecal streptococci, but micrococci are hard to see. In patients who have started treatment with a penicillin or cephalosporin, coliforms appear elongated as cell wall synthesis is disrupted. *Yeast* cells are sometimes difficult to distinguish from leucocytes but they tend to have variable cell size and cell budding is a distinguishing feature (Figure 2.1b).

The interpretation of urine microscopy findings needs to take into account the method of urine collection and the age and sex of the patient. The presence of more than 10 WBCs μl^{-1} in a freshly voided uncentrifuged MSU or clean-catch sample should be regarded as abnormal, with the exception of infant girls in whom a count of twice this is often found. On bag urine samples higher numbers of WBCs are common even in the absence of vulvitis or balanitis (Littlewood, 1971). A helpful clue in examining any voided urine is the presence or absence of squamous cells. These are always derived from the external genitalia (the uroepithelium is transitional) and indicate that a urine sample is contaminated. Bag samples from infants give a 10% false-positive rate on urine culture alone, and here prompt microscopy is especially helpful in deciding whether to discard the specimen in favour of a suprapubic aspiration.

Culture

Urine is a good culture medium and at room temperature most coliform bacteria will self-replicate about every 20 min. Because in voided urine the quantification of bacteriuria is important in making a diagnosis of infection, it is recommended that the urine is plated out for culture within 1 hour. This poses no difficulty within a hospital during the working day but in general practice or out of hours alternative plans are needed. Refrigerating these samples to 4°C inhibits bacterial growth and allows the culturing to be deferred for several hours. The drawback of this is that the result is also delayed and one never really knows whether all the bacteria in the sample have been similarly growth retarded. The dip slide (Oxoid or Uricult) overcomes this problem.

The dip slide consists of a sterile universal container with a culture plate mounted within the screw-on cap (Figure 2.2). MacConkey's agar is used on one side of the plate and on the reverse the Oxoid dip slide uses cystine-lactose-electrolyte-deficient medium whereas Uricult has either this or a nutrient agar. The two types were shown to give similar results during a screening study for bacteriuria in schoolgirls (Edwards *et al.*, 1975). The plate is immersed in the urine making sure that all of the surface is equally wetted, then withdrawn and screwed back into its universal container. Incubation will begin at room temperature and the dip slide is sufficiently robust to be posted to a laboratory if necessary. This is useful for children with recurrent urinary infection who can be shown how to inoculate a dip slide at home using the 'dip stream' technique (voiding directly over the agar plate). If symptomatic they may then take a single dose of antibiotic and post the dip slide to their doctor. After incubation for 24 h at 37°C the numbers of colonies can be read with precision by

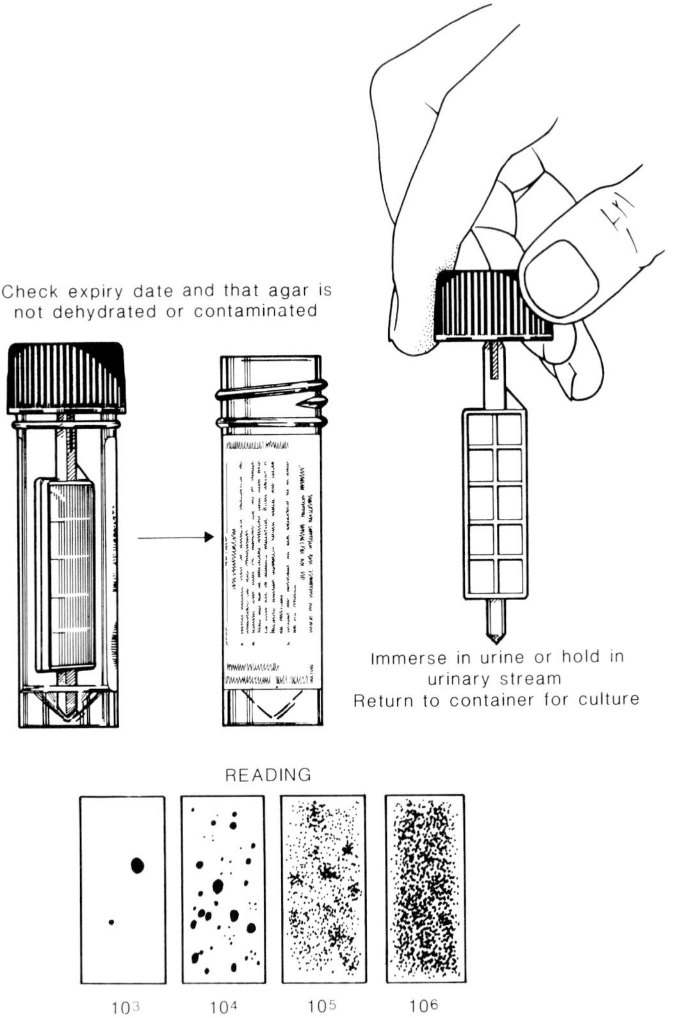

Figure 2.2 The Oxoid dip slide

inspecting the plate. One can usually recognize whether there is a
single strain present, in which case the colonies are of similar size, or
whether there is a mixture of species. Subsequently the laboratory
can define the organism involved and perform antibiotic sensitivity
tests if necessary.

It should be noted, however, that when the dip slides are used to
culture bag urine samples from infants, especially girls, a false-

positive rate of 10% can be expected. This highlights the need for urine microscopy so that those samples containing squamous cells can be discarded from culture and the collection repeated or alternative methods used.

Laboratories use a variety of plating and culturing techniques from which the viable colony count per ml of urine can be gauged. The pioneering work of Kass (1956) showed that in adults a colony count of $> 10^5$ ml^{-1} of an organism in pure culture gave convincing evidence of bladder urine infection. This holds true in paediatric practice as long as the urine sample is midstream. In a suprapubic aspirate any growth is significant.

The organisms usually grown from infected children are *Escherichia coli* ($>90\%$), *Streptococcus faecalis*, *Klebsiella* species and staphylococci. *Proteus* is frequently cultured from boys with balanitis, but is rarely a true bladder pathogen. All these are aerobic bacteria and apart from temperature and nutrient have no special culture needs. In hospital patients, and especially those with hydrodynamically abnormal urinary tracts, less common bacterial species are found. To identify anaerobes or fastidious organisms additional laboratory procedures are required. Moreover the clinician should be aware that viral infections of the urinary tract occur; adenovirus 11 and cytomegalovirus have been reported (Mufson *et al.*, 1971; Davies *et al.*, 1979). If a child with symptoms of acute cystitis who has not received antibiotic has negative, routine aerobic urine cultures it is worth discussing further investigation with the microbiologist.

References

Davies, J. G., Taylor, C. M., White, R. H. R. *et al.* (1979) Cytomegalovirus infection associated with lower urinary tract symptoms. *British Medical Journal*, **1**, 1120

Edwards, B., White, R. H. R., Maxted, H. *et al.* (1975) Screening methods for covert bacteriuria in school girls. *British Medical Journal*, **1**, 463–467

Fairley, K. F. and Birch, D. F. (1982) Hematuria: a simple method for identifying glomerular bleeding. *Kidney International*, **21**, 105–108

Kass, E. H. (1956) Asymptomatic infections of the urinary tract. *Transactions of the Association of American Physicians*, **64**, 56–63

Littlewood, J. M. (1971) White cells and bacteria in voiding urine of healthy newborns. *Archives of Disease in Childhood*, **46**, 167–172

Mufson, M. A., Zollar, I. M., Mankad, V. *et al.* (1971) Adenovirus infections in acute hemorrhagic cystitis: a study in 25 children. *American Journal of Disease in Children*, **121**, 281–285

Rizzoni, G., Braggion, F., Grando, F. *et al.* (1984) Detection of glomerular and non-glomerular bleeding. *Journal of Pediatrics*, **104**, 161

Robins, D. G., White, R. H. R., Rogers, K. B. and Osman, M. S. (1975) Urine microscopy as an aid to detection of bacteriuria. *Lancet*, **i**, 476–477

Chapter 3

Urinalysis

Introduction

Long before Galileo developed the microscope, physicians have peered at urine samples in the hope of diagnostic inspiration. Urinary colour and odour can still give useful clues to systemic disease. Red urine may indicate haematuria but free haemoglobin, myoglobin and various food dyes can give similar appearances, and a red colour which develops on exposure to the air suggests the presence of porphyrins. The haematuria of glomerulonephritis usually appears as an opalescent sample with a reddy brown colour due to the decomposition of haemoglobin. Moreover in nephritis blood is uniformly mixed with the urine, whereas in haemorrhagic cystitis, for example, haematuria is more evident at the end of the urinary stream (terminal haematuria). Urates are orange in colour, and a dark-orange urate stain on a neonate's nappy should not be confused with haematuria. Very rarely one sees the brown-black urine of alcaptonuria or tyrosinosis, or the blue discoloration of some disorders of tryptophan metabolism.

Cloudy urine may be an indication of leucocyturia but is also caused by oxalate and phosphate aggregates. Adding a drop of acetic acid or rewarming the specimen respectively will redissolve these crystals to allow microscopy to be performed. In urinary tract infection urea-splitting organisms will give fresh urine a fishy, ammoniacal smell. Urine-soaked skin eventually develops this odour so that children with incontinence are often suspected, perhaps incorrectly, of having urinary infection.

Today there is a growing range of dipsticks which give powerful chemical analysis into the hands of the clinician at the bedside or in the outpatient clinic. Here we give a review of those most relevant to renal disease. With all of these reagents it is important to store them appropriately, ensure that they are within their expiry date, and to follow exactly the manufacturer's instructions.

Specific gravity

Where precise information on urine osmolality is needed it should be measured accurately by the depression of freezing point (see Chapter 6). In the absence of proteinuria or glycosuria there is broad agreement between osmolality and specific gravity (Leech and Penney, 1987). In infants particularly the volume of urine obtained at any time is small and it is therefore impractical to use a hydrometer. A refractometer (American Optical Company, or Atago, Uricon) is a valuable device which uses only one drop of urine and gives a good indication of specific gravity. The instrument is robust, and although rather expensive to purchase lasts a lifetime and has no running costs (Figure 3.1). It is ideal for an intensive care or neonatal ward.

In health, specific gravity ranges from 1.002 to 1.035; these figures correlating with an osmolality of 50 and 1300 mosmol kg^{-1} respectively.

More recently specific gravity has become measurable with a dipstick (Multistix SG, Ames). This test gives a colour change depending on the ionic concentration of the test solution. A small adjustment has to be made for urine with pH of more than 6.5; however, it is said by the manufacturers to give a good correlation with refractometer results.

pH

Reagent strips using methyl red and bromthymol blue permit a wide

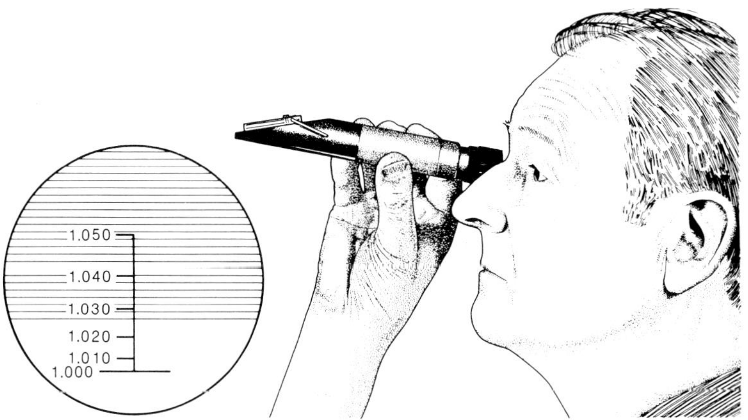

Figure 3.1 The Atago refractometer

colour range from pH 5 to 8.5. The test is not influenced by the normal buffers in the urine. Only freshly voided urine should be tested as bacterial contamination will alter pH. This is a good screening measure of urinary pH, but in the evaluation of metabolic acidosis the urinary pH should be confirmed with a hydrogen ion electrode.

Proteinuria

For details about Albustix (Ames) see pages 20–21.

Haematuria

Haemastix (Ames) relies on the peroxidase-like activity of haemoglobin to catalyse the reaction of a hydroperoxide on tetramethylbenzidine to give a green-blue colour. Myoglobin also catalyses this reaction. The antioxidant ascorbic acid reduces the sensitivity of the test. The test is capable of detecting as little as $150\,\mu g\,l^{-1}$ of free haemoglobin (less than 20 intact red cells μl^{-1}). Because the test is so sensitive a negative result can be taken to exclude significant haematuria. Even in a dilute urine specimen in which erythrocytes have lysed it is quite possible to have a positive Haemastix test and not see any red cells on routine microscopy. If careful microscopy of centrifuged urine fails to identify red cells the possibility of haemoglobinuria or myoglobinuria is raised. Urine electrophoresis distinguishes between these two.

Parents can be easily instructed to test their child's urine and record the results. This is useful information in the patient with *isolated* microscopic haematuria; persistent haematuria over a period of 6 months is a reasonable indication for a renal biopsy whereas intermittent haematuria requires monitoring only (see Appendix 2).

Nitrite

There have been several attempts to provide a chemical test for identifying urinary tract infection. So far none has succeeded in completely replacing conventional microbiological techniques. The nitrite test was developed from a test for bacterial contamination of the public water supply. It uses the observation that certain microorganisms reduce the nitrate, present in ground water as in urine, to nitrite. Urine is normally nitrite free. Gram-negative coliform bacilli and *Strep. faecalis*, which are responsible for at least nine out of ten urinary tract infections, are capable of reducing nitrate. *Staphylococcus albus* and micrococci give variable results.

The test strip contains para-arsanilic acid which reacts with the nitrite to produce a diazonium compound which is then coupled to 3-hydroxy-1,2,3,4-tetrahydrobenzo (h)-quinolin-3-ol to produce an azo dye. This reaction is highly specific and any pink coloration is an indication of nitrite.

Urine containing nitrate has to be in contact with the bacteria for some time for the nitrite to be produced. If a contaminated urine sample is left to stand the nitrite test will become positive and therefore it is essential that only freshly voided samples are tested. With this proviso false-positive diagnoses of urinary tract infection are uncommon but false negatives occur. Unfortunately this appears to be particularly the case with symptomatic patients who, perhaps because of frequency of micturition, do not give time for the urinary nitrate to be converted in the bladder (Smellie, 1983; Powell, McCredie and Ritchie, 1987).

Ketones

Children who are fasted or febrile readily excrete ketones in their urine. However, in the investigation of a patient with a metabolic acidosis it is valuable to document the presence of ketones in the urine, especially if there is an increased anion gap. Strip reagents contain sodium nitroprusside in a buffer, which reacts with aceto acetic acid to give a pink or maroon colour. The reagent strip will pick up large quantities of phenylketones such as in phenylketonuria and it will react with bromosulphthalein (BSP) used in the BSP excretion test.

Glucose

Two different tests are available: Clinitest (Ames), which detects all reducing sugars, and a glucose oxidase-impregnated dipstick, Diastix (Ames), which is specific for glucose. The former consists of a tablet containing copper sulphate and sodium hydroxide. Reducing sugars convert the copper sulphate to cuprous oxide changing the colour of the solution from blue to orange. The test will detect lactose (for example in some newborn milk-fed infants), fructose, galactose, pentose and reducing substances such as ascorbic acid. The glucose-specific reagent strip uses glucose oxidase to catalyse the formation of gluconic acid and hydrogen peroxide from glucose. The hydrogen peroxide then reacts with potassium iodide, the reaction being catalysed by inclusion of a peroxidase, and a green colour results. A concentration of 5.5 mmol 1^{-1} of glucose is detectable. This concentration is higher than the physiological concentration of glucose in the urine; however, the test is more sensitive than Clinitest. High doses of salicylate may give a falsely reduced reading with Diastix and the presence of ketones may reduce colour development of the strip. If a urine sample is positive with Clinitest, but negative with Diastix, it suggests that the reducing substance is other than glucose and in infancy it is important, therefore, to test for galactose and other sugars specifically.

A reduction of the normal concentration of urinary glucose can be caused by bacterial metabolism, a situation analogous to the lowering of cerebrospinal fluid glucose in meningitis (Schersten, Fritz and Kohler, 1967). Uriglox (Warner) is a highly sensitive glucose oxidase strip designed to detect concentrations as low as $100\,\mu\mathrm{mol\,l^{-1}}$ $(2\,\mathrm{mg\,dl^{-1}})$; a level below this in an early morning sample is suggestive of urinary tract infection. This test has been overtaken by the nitrite test.

Leucocytes

Cytur-Test (BCL) measures leucocyte esterases and therefore gives an indication of the presence of leucocytes. These esterases cleave an indoxyl ester and the free indoxyl is then oxidized to indigo blue. The test is sensitive enough to be positive for a urine containing more than 10 leucocytes $\mu\mathrm{l^{-1}}$ and will show positivity after the cells have lysed. There is general agreement claimed between this strip reagent and microscopy. Nevertheless this test is still very much dependent on the method of urine collection and its only advantage over conventional microscopy is capital cost. It may therefore find a place in primary health care, but the versatility and additional information obtained by microscopy cannot be replaced by this.

References

Leech, S. and Penney, M. D. (1987) Correlation of specific gravity and osmolality of urines in neonates and adults. *Archives of Disease in Childhood*, **62**, 671–673

Powell, H. R., McCredie, D. A. and Ritchie, M. A. (1987) Urinary nitrite in symptomatic and asymptomatic urinary infection. *Archives of Disease in Childhood*, **62**, 138–140

Schersten, B., Fritz, H. and Kohler, L. (1967) Subnormal concentrations of urinary glucose as a sign of urinary tract infection in children. *Acta Paediatrica Scandinavica*, Suppl. **177**, 54–56

Smellie, J. (1983) The nitrite test for bacteruria. In *Focus on Urine Analysis*, The Medicine Publishing Foundation, Oxford, pp. 15–17

Chapter 4

Proteinuria

Introduction

The urine of healthy people contains a very small quantity of protein, and an increase in protein excretion is one of the most sensitive indicators of renal pathology. Urinary proteins are derived from the plasma as well as being actively secreted by the tubule. Albumin is the most prevalent of the plasma proteins found in the urine and accounts for 10% of the total. Secretory IgA and the high molecular weight uromucoid, Tamm–Horsfall protein, are secreted by the tubule itself. The latter, which is produced in the ascending limb of the loop of Henle and probably restricts water efflux at this site, contributes approximately 40% of the normal urinary protein. It also forms the matrix of many urinary casts.

The glomerular capillary wall allows water, electrolytes and small molecules to pass freely into the urinary space but retains larger ones, a process explained as 'molecular sieving'. For molecules with a radius of up to 20 Å the sieving coefficient can be regarded as 100%.

Albumin, the most abundant and one of the smaller plasma proteins, has a molecular radius of 35 Å which markedly restricts its passage across the basement membrane. Moreover it is negatively charged and is repelled from the capillary wall by the high density of polyanionic mucoproteins on the surface of endothelial and epithelial cells. The clearance of albumin into the fluid of the proximal tubule is 0.04% that of inulin (sieving coefficient 0.04%). The albumin which does escape into the tubular fluid is extensively recovered by pinocytosis and catabolized by tubular epithelium; only 1% of the filtered load finally appears in bladder urine. However, the capacity of the tubule to recover filtered protein is close to the maximum achievable so that a small increase in protein leakage from the glomerulus can give rise to a marked increase in proteinuria. In this way there is a far greater potential for glomerular, rather than tubular lesions to cause heavy proteinuria.

Tubular damage itself may be associated with an increased loss of *normally* filtered small plasma proteins because of their impaired recovery. An example of such a protein is B_2 microglobulin, a product of lymphocytes and related to the HLA (human leucocyte antigen) antigen complex, which has a molecular radius of 16 Å. Increased urinary clearance of B_2 microglobulin can be used as a marker of tubular dysfunction and tubulo-interstitial disease (Portman, Kissane and Robson, 1986). The excretion of very small *abnormal* plasma proteins by otherwise normal kidneys can occur, such as Bence Jones proteinuria in myeloma, a disorder of dismissible rarity in childhood.

Although the pattern of different proteins excreted in renal disease can be useful diagnostically, this is largely a tool for research or specialist centres. Too much emphasis has been placed, for example, on 'protein selectivity' in childhood nephrotic syndrome. In this test the clearance of a larger protein (IgG) and a smaller one (transferrin) is compared. A selective proteinuria, in which the IgG/transferrin clearance ratio is $<10\%$, is typical of the minimal change nephrotic syndrome whereas poorly selective proteinuria suggests a destructive glomerular lesion. In practice the quickest way to identify the child with minimal change is a trial of steroid treatment. Moreover there are some unexpected exceptions, such as high selectivity in the Finnish type of congenital nephrotic syndrome (Huttunen *et al.*, 1980), and because of the confusion that sometimes arises this test is best forgotten.

The physiological range of total protein excretion is constant above 3 years of age, and the sex difference inconsequential. However, albumin excretion, in $mg^{-1} day^{-1}$ per m^2 body surface area (BSA), shows a shallow rise between the ages of 4 and 16 years (Davies *et al.*, 1984). In infants excretion rates expressed as a ratio of urinary creatinine are higher (Barratt, McLaine and Soothill, 1970), particularly in the pre-term. Healthy individuals show a considerable day-to-day variation within the normal range. The excretion of up to 10 times the upper limit of normal is generally regarded as 'moderate' proteinuria in which disturbances of plasma albumin are not expected. Protein excretion rates greater than this are regarded as 'heavy' and, when this reaches 20 or more times the normal, clinically relevant disturbances of plasma proteins occur.

Methods of protein measurement

Albustix (Ames)
These reagent strips use a dye-binding technique, and rely on the observation that bound dye (tetrabromphenol blue) has a different absorption maximum and thus a colour change is seen. Although

Table 4.1 Concentration of protein detectable by Albustix

Albustix reading	Protein concentration (mg l^{-1})
Trace	50–200
+	300
+ +	1 000
+ + +	3 000
+ + + +	10 000

not specific for albumin, this protein binds more avidly than others. As a clinical tool these dipsticks are cheap, reliable and give instant semi-quantitative results. One should note that a strongly alkaline urine may give a false-positive result with Albustix and that some specific proteins, such as Bence Jones protein, fail to react. The concentration of protein detectable by Albustix is shown in Table 4.1.

Albustix is used to identify moderate or severe proteinuria such as that seen in patients with nephritis or a nephrotic syndrome. It should be noted that a subtle increase in protein excretion rate, so-called microproteinuria, is undetectable by Albustix. Microproteinuria is seen in some patients who have a marked reduction of renal mass or diabetes mellitus. When consistent this observation implies that glomerular sclerosis is taking place; proteinuria will then worsen and glomerular filtration rate (GFR) decline. In these circumstances more precise quantification is needed (see the clinical example in Figure 4.1).

Laboratory methods
There are several methods used for the measurement of either total or individual proteins in urine.

For measuring total protein the *Biuret* method has a long tradition in many laboratories. Peptides form a coloured complex with copper (copper sulphate) in an alkaline solution (sodium hydroxide). Absorption is then measured at 540 nm and compared with standard curves. The method loses accuracy at low protein concentrations, and for this reason alternatives are needed. The *Coomassie blue* dye-binding technique (Bradford, 1976), which is simple, inexpensive and lends itself to automation, gives superior precision at low concentrations and is able to quantify microproteinuria.

Albumin can be measured accurately by radioimmunoassay (RIA) (Keen and Chlouverakis, 1963), ELISA (Fielding, Price and Houlton, 1983) or immunodiffusion techniques at concentrations as

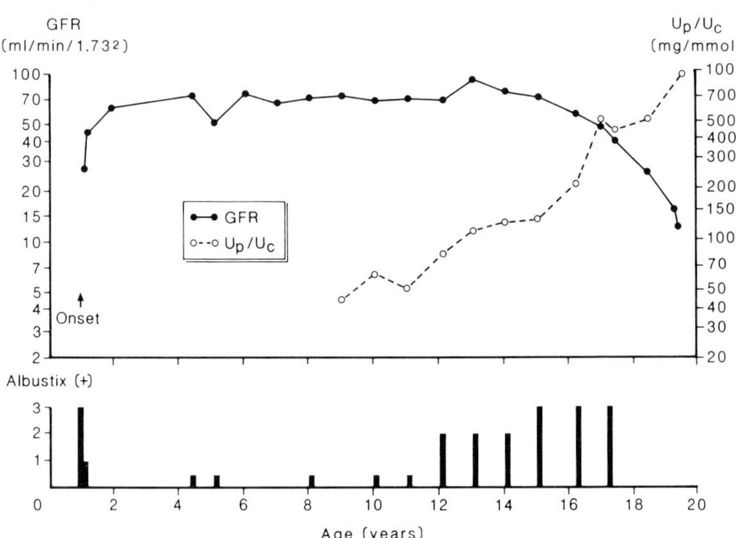

Figure 4.1 Monitoring GFR and urinary protein excretion. The patient illustrated had the haemolytic uraemic syndrome in infancy and made a good initial recovery. The late decline in renal function was anticipated by worsening proteinuria. Renal function flow charts are available from the Children's Hospital, Birmingham

low as $10\,\mathrm{mg\,l^{-1}}$. There is a vogue for urinary albumin testing and new kits using latex particle agglutination inhibition are being marketed. However, in the majority of renal diseases changes in albumin excretion mirror those of total protein so that there is little value in adopting more costly albumin assays.

Early morning urine samples

Proteinuria increases physiologically with upright posture and physical activity. Moreover, surgery, trauma and pyrexia commonly give rise to a transient increase in urinary protein. Renal pathology is indicated by a *consistent* increase in urinary protein excretion. About 15% of patients with orthostatic or postural proteinuria demonstrate a persistently raised daytime protein excretion; however, long-term studies confirm that this anomaly may be regarded as a benign disorder. Therefore in order to avoid false-positive results and anxiety for patients it is essential to test urine formed while the patient was supine. This can be quantified in either a timed overnight urine collection or derived more simply as a protein/

creatinine ratio on an early morning urine (EMU) sample. *There is no place for 24-hour urine collections to document the protein excretion rate in everyday paediatric practice.*

It is an easy matter to ask outpatients to bring an EMU sample with them to the clinic and this is the method preferred. Children are instructed to void to completion immediately before bedtime on the night before the EMU collection. Nocturia or nocturnal enuresis does not interfere as the test does not require a timed sample. As soon as the child wakes in the morning urine is collected in a universal container. If after dipstick testing in the outpatient clinic precise laboratory quantification of protein excretion is needed, for example in monitoring children with chronic renal failure or reduced renal mass, it can be requested on the same sample.

Just as testing an EMU sample avoids any confusion caused by postural or exercise-induced proteinuria, so patients with steroid-responsive (minimal change) nephrotic syndrome, monitoring their urine at home with Albustix, should be warned not to test the urine at other times in the day as the finding of the occasional 1 or 2+ proteinuria creates unnecessary anxiety. By testing an EMU sample daily they get clear evidence of any new relapse. Most paediatric nephrologists define a relapse as 3+ proteinuria for 3 consecutive days, and this usually gives enough time to start treatment and control the condition before oedema appears.

Quantification of protein excretion

For practical purposes creatinine excretion is constant in an individual, and is proportional to muscle mass. Therefore by relating the urinary protein to urinary creatinine concentration one derives a ratio which is factored for both time and body size. This correlates closely with a measured protein excretion rate (Elises *et al.*, 1988), the latter being expressed as mass of protein per time per BSA of the child. For timed total protein measurements the usually quoted upper limit of normal is $4\,\mathrm{mg\,h^{-1}}$ per $\mathrm{m^2}$, a figure adopted by the International Study of Kidney Disease in Childhood.

Using the Coomassie blue *total protein* measurement Elises *et al.* (1988) have shown that in children over 2 years the upper limit of normal EMU protein/creatinine ratio is $20\,\mathrm{mg\,mmol^{-1}}$.

The *albumin*/creatinine ratio appears to depend somewhat on the method of analysis. Davies *et al.* (1984) regard the upper limit to be $1.7\,\mathrm{mg\,mmol^{-1}}$, and Elises *et al.* (1988) $3\,\mathrm{mg\,mmol^{-1}}$. (To convert to $\mathrm{mg\,mg^{-1}}$ creatinine divide by 113.) For infants it is best to refer to Barratt, McLaine and Soothill (1970) who have standardized excretion against body weight.

Summary

- Persistent proteinuria is a strong indicator of clinically significant renal disease.
- Always test EMU samples to avoid confusion with orthostatic proteinuria.
- Albustix is a convenient method of screening for moderate or severe proteinuria.
- For precise quantification of protein excretion use the EMU protein/creatinine or albumin/creatinine ratio.

References

Barratt, T. M., McLaine, P. N. and Soothill, J. F. (1970) Albumin excretion as a measure of glomerular dysfunction in children. *Archives of Disease in Childhood*, **45**, 496–501

Bradford, M. M. (1976) A rapid and sensitive method for quantitation of microgram quantities of protein utilizing the principle of protein binding. *Analytical Biochemistry*, **72**, 248–254

Davies, A. G., Postlethwaite, R. J., Price, D. A. *et al.* (1984) Urinary albumin excretion in school children. *Archives of Disease in Childhood*, **59**, 625–630

Elises, J. S., Griffiths, P. D., Hocking, M. D. *et al.* (1988) Simplified quantification of urinary protein excretion in children. *Clinical Nephrology*, **30**, 225–229

Fielding, B. A., Price, D. A. and Houlton, C. A. (1983) Enzyme immunoassay for urinary albumin. *Clinical Chemistry*, **29**, 355–357

Huttunen, N. P., Vehaskari, M., Viikari, M. and Laipio, M. L. (1980) Proteinuria in the congenital nephrotic syndrome of the Finnish type. *Clinical Nephrology*, **13**, 12–19

Keen, H. and Chlouverakis, C. (1963) An immunoassay method for urinary albumin at low concentration. *Lancet*, **ii**, 913–914

Portman, R. J., Kissane, J. M. and Robson, A. M. (1986) Use of B_2 microglobulin to diagnose tubulo-interstitial renal disease in children. *Kidney International*, **30**, 91–98

Chapter 5

Glomerular filtration rate and plasma creatinine

Introduction

The kidney controls the volume and composition of extracellular fluid by two interlocking processes, glomerular filtration and tubular reabsorption. Both in health, and in the majority of renal diseases, the rate of glomerular filtration is regulated to match the tubules' ability to handle salt and water. For this reason the measurement of glomerular filtration rate (GFR) gives the clinician a useful indication of overall renal, not just glomerular performance.

The kidneys receive approximately 20% of the cardiac output, which in the 70-kg adult is approximately 1 litre of blood or 600 ml plasma min^{-1}. The vascular anatomy of the kidney is such that the arterial blood is almost entirely delivered to the glomeruli, the vascular supply to the tubules being taken from the glomerular efferent arterioles. Thus the 600 ml plasma min^{-1} (effective renal plasma flow, ERPF) are presented to the glomeruli. One hundred and twenty-five ml of this fluid are filtered across the capillary membrane and emerge into the urinary space within Bowman's capsule. Ninety-nine per cent of it will then be reabsorbed by the tubule and returned to the circulation. If we assume that the plasma volume in this subject is 3.5 litres, it can be calculated that the plasma water is entirely filtered and reabsorbed every 24 minutes!

In theory, filtration depends on the systemic arterial blood pressure, renal blood flow, the surface area of the glomerular capillary walls and the permeability of the filtration membrane. Autoregulation takes place so that in practice the GFR remains constant over a wide range of systemic blood pressure. Some species exhibit considerable fluctuations in GFR depending on their physical activity and their fed or fasted state. Perhaps because of the constancy of our lifestyle humans demonstrate only minor diurnal variation in GFR.

Paediatric considerations

In normal individuals the rate of glomerular filtration is related to

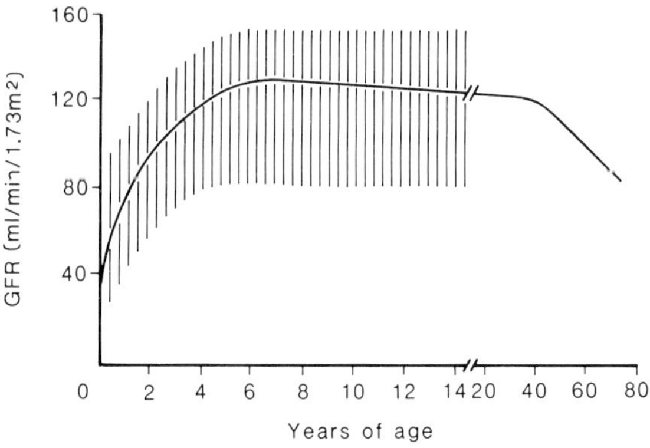

Figure 5.1 The physiological change of GFR/body surface area with age

body size. It is convenient that in human beings the GFR (ml min^{-1}) is directly proportional to body surface area (BSA) from the age of 3 years until middle adult life. For this reason GFR is conventionally expressed in ml min^{-1} per 1.73 m^2, the suffix being the 'average' adult BSA. In clinical practice monitoring the GFR of a growing child above 3 years of age, it is imperative to correct for BSA and the corrective figures will accurately represent any functional change in the patient. The relationship with BSA does not hold good in the period below 3 years of age during which renal function undergoes a process of maturation (McCrory, 1972) and this reduces precision (Figure 5.1). It has been argued that in comparing the GFR of infants it is better to standardize for body weight (Coultard and Hey, 1984). Nevertheless for patients below 3 years most nephrologists still correct for BSA and, with Figure 5.1 in mind, make an enlightened guess as to whether renal function is markedly abnormal or not. With sequential observations in this age-group, one can usually judge whether the change in BSA-corrected GFR matches the normal curve.

Clinical relevance of GFR measurement

Glomeruli once destroyed cannot be regenerated. However, in any renal disease the less badly affected glomeruli have a marked capacity for both functional and anatomical compensatory hypertrophy. This has important implications for use of GFR measurements in clinical practice. A focal lesion of the kidney can destroy a lot of tissue without causing any significant fall in GFR. Alternatively by the time a focal lesion *has* caused renal impairment parenchymal damage will have occurred on a large scale. A good clinical example of this problem is the coarse renal scarring of reflux nephropathy (chronic pyelonephritis) which is the commonest renal lesion in childhood. If a patient is found to have an area of scarring in one kidney, the measurement of overall GFR will be normal; indeed there is no place for the measurement of total GFR in such children. On the other hand, if in a child with renal impairment the underlying diagnosis is found to be renal scarring it will certainly be bilateral and extensive (White and Taylor, 1984). It is in the former example of unilateral damage that the estimation of individual kidney GFR from a renogram is valuable (see below).

With diffuse renal disease it has often been observed that the most profound reduction in GFR is seen in tubulo-interstitial lesions rather than glomerular ones. This is probably because the normal autoregulation of GFR, which is effected by the tubule, is disturbed. As an oversimplification a patient with normal-size kidneys, mild proteinuria and a profound fall in GFR is likely to have tubulo-interstitial disease. By contrast a patient with glomerulonephritis has heavy proteinuria and the GFR falls as a late event.

The concept of clearance

It is relatively easy to visualize the net movement of water from the plasma across the glomerular basement membrane into the urinary space, the volume cleared in a given time being the GFR. However, there is no direct way of measuring the filtrate. It is assumed that small molecules cross the glomerular membrane as freely as water. If such a substance is biologically inert, precisely measurable in blood and urine and is neither reabsorbed nor excreted by the tubule, its clearance from blood into the urine can be calculated as follows:

Amount cleared = urine volume × urinary concentration (UV).

However, the amount cleared will be directly proportional to the concentration of the substance in the plasma, that is the amount presented to the glomerulus. The rate of clearance is therefore expressed in the time-honoured formula UV/P where U is the urine concentration, V is the urine volume and P is the plasma concentration of the substance. By this calculation we obtain the *volume* of plasma which contains the amount of the test substance which was cleared in a given time.

The gold standard for measurement of GFR is *inulin clearance*. This inert sugar is infused to give a constant plasma concentration. Timed urine collections are made and this may require bladder catheterization for accuracy. This is a complex procedure for the patient, clinician and laboratory, and it is therefore only used as a research investigation. The following section refers to more practical methods which have either directly or indirectly been equated to inulin clearance.

[51]Chromium-edetic acid clearance

This stable radionuclide which has a molecular weight of 344 meets all the requirements of a marker for clearance studies. The [51]chromium label remains firmly attached to the chelate, the compound exhibits minimal protein binding and is freely filtered at the glomerulus with negligible tubular handling thereafter. As with inulin formal clearance studies can be performed with a continuous infusion to give a constant plasma concentration, and with accurately timed urine samples. This too is a research tool, the more practical ^{51}Cr-EDTA (edetic acid) slope clearance method being favoured in clinical practice (Chantler and Barratt, 1972).

Theory of slope clearance method
After an intravenous bolus injection the chelate quickly equilibrates with the extracellular fluid (ECF). Experience shows that this process is complete within 90 min. After that time the plasma activity falls exponentially as the chelate is excreted by glomerular filtration, and the GFR can be predicted from the slope of the plasma activity curve (Figure 5.2). The formula used to predict clearance was derived from studies by Newman, Bordley and Winternitz (1944) using mannitol as the marker substance:

$$\text{Clearance} = \frac{\text{theoretical volume of distribution} \times 0.693}{\text{half time}}.$$

Clearly some of the assumptions in the slope clearance theory are oversimplified. There is not instant mixing of the chelate into its theoretical volume of distribution, and in the first minutes after injection a higher concentration is presented to the glomerulus and more is cleared. The estimated plasma concentration at time zero is therefore an underestimate. The theoretical volume of distribution is calculated by dividing the estimated plasma concentration at time zero by the dose injected, and this volume is therefore overestimated.

Just as errors accrue as the chelate equilibrates from vascular to extravascular compartments, so in the later phase the concentration in the plasma is lower than that in the interstitial fluid because of glomerular clearance. Attempts have been made to adjust for the latter using double exponential analysis. This gives a closer estimate of the true GFR but the method requires analysis of the initial phase

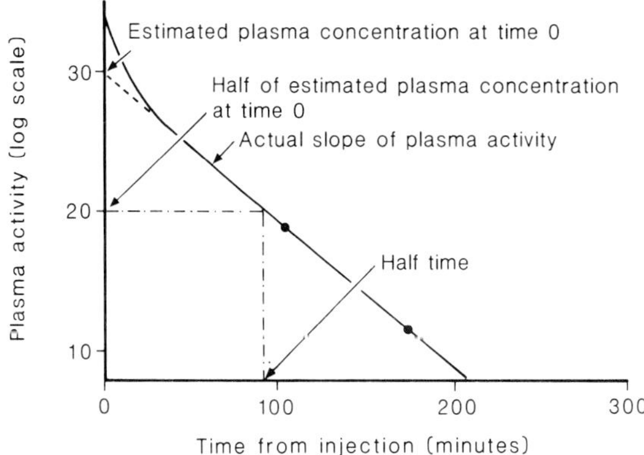

Figure 5.2 Plasma activity curve following bolus injection of ^{51}Cr-EDTA

of the plasma activity curve and therefore needs multiple blood samples.

The reliability of the monoexponential estimate of GFR using ^{51}Cr-EDTA has been carefully evaluated (Chantler and Barratt, 1972). The linear part of the slope can be accurately plotted from the plasma activity of two blood samples, the first at 120 min and the second at 240 min or later if renal function is impaired. Additional samples make only a very small improvement to the accuracy of the slope. ^{51}Cr-EDTA has a renal clearance which is 5% less than inulin and it is conventional to multiply by a correction factor of 1.05. Because single exponential analysis overestimates simultaneously performed formal clearances of ^{51}Cr-EDTA, a further correction of 0.77 is required (Chantler *et al.*, 1969). In normally hydrated individuals repeated measurements of ^{51}Cr-EDTA slope clearance by this method have been shown to have a coefficient of variation of less than 4% (Chantler and Barratt, 1972).

[51]Cr-EDTA slope clearance: practical aspects
This method cannot be applied to children who are either dehydrated or oedematous. ^{51}Cr-EDTA, a beta emitter with a half-life of 28 days, is measured in biological tissues by a scintillation counter. The radiation exposure from a ^{51}Cr-EDTA clearance is minute, being estimated as less than 1 week of natural background radiation. Clearly the urinary epithelium is the target organ for most of this radiation and by inducing a vigorous diuresis and encouraging frequent bladder emptying this exposure is minimized.

First, the child's height and weight are accurately measured so that BSA can be deduced. Although many still use the formula of

Du Bois and Du Bois (1916), that of Haycock, Schwartz and Wisotsky (1978) is superior. The radiopharmacy prepares a sterile weighed dose containing $1.0\,\mu\text{Ci kg}^{-1}$ body weight. This is injected into a well-sited intravenous cannula. The cannula must not have side ports in which the chelate can pool and the dose should be flushed through by injection of 10 ml of saline. The syringe containing the chelate is returned to the pharmacy for reweighing. The cannula is removed and also taken for counting to ensure that the dose has been completely delivered. One ml of blood is drawn from a contralateral forearm vein at approximately 120 min. The exact time is recorded. The timing of the second sample is chosen to give a clear separation between the two measurements. If the patient is expected to have normal renal function the second sample may be drawn at 3 h after injection, but with renal failure it should be extended to 6 h.

Estimation of individual kidney GFR

With focal or unilateral renal disease it is often necessary to have some measure of the function of an individual kidney. Formal clearance studies using the formula UV/P are possible if the child has ureterostomies or if the upper tracts are cannulated. In the intact child external pressure applied to the side of the abdomen is able to occlude a ureter as it crosses the pelvic brim, and bladder urine can be collected from the contralateral kidney. However, this method had been superseded by isotope renography.

^{99m}Technetium-DTPA (diethylenetriamine pentacetic acid) is a gamma emitter and lends itself to renal imaging (see Chapter 11). This radiopharmaceutical is handled in the kidney almost identically to ^{51}Cr-EDTA, and although some of the preparations pose variable protein binding, and therefore underestimate clearance, an excellent agreement between simultaneously performed clearances of ^{51}Cr-EDTA and Pentetate (Amersham International) has recently been shown in children (Griffiths *et al.*, 1988).

The overall GFR is estimated by ^{99m}Tc-DTPA slope clearance in the same way as for ^{51}Cr-EDTA. This is then divided in proportion to the activity arising from each kidney in the second phase of the renogram to give a figure of GFR for each (Piepsz *et al.*, 1978; Kainer *et al.*, 1979).

If the overall GFR is known from some other method, the differential uptake between kidneys of either iodine-labelled hippuran, which is otherwise used to measure effective renal plasma flow, or ^{99m}Tc-dimercaptosuccinic acid (DMSA), which is for imaging renal parenchyma, will also permit an estimate of individual kidney function.

Methods using plasma creatinine

The clearance of endogenous creatinine was for a long time the mainstay of GFR estimation. There are, however, a number of drawbacks, some of which are particularly relevant to paediatric practice. First, a formal clearance study requires complete and timed urine collection. This is a near impossibility in small children or in any patient with a hydrodynamically abnormal urinary tract, e.g. vesico-ureteric reflux (VUR) (Winterborn, Beetham and White, 1977).

Although alternatives exist creatinine is usually measured by the Jaffé reaction. This is subject to interference from non-creatinine chromogens normally present in the plasma, various antibiotics, and a compound occurring in jaundice. Unless care is taken, such as applying reaction-rate methods to avoid reading non-creatinine chromogens, the Jaffé reaction lacks precision at low creatinine concentrations. As the plasma creatinine concentration in small children is lower than in adults any overestimation, appearing in the denominator of the UV/P calculation, gives a falsely low clearance.

Creatinine is to some extent secreted by the renal tubules, and this is more marked in chronic renal failure so that creatinine overestimates true GFR. Moreover, a small increase in plasma creatinine can be observed after vigorous muscular exertion or after ingesting meat.

Creatinine has a molecular weight of 113 and is derived from the non-enzymatic degradation of creatine phosphate within muscle. The daily urinary excretion has been shown to be proportional to weight and, at a pinch, body weight is proportional to the cube of height and surface area to the square of height. The clearance formula can be rationalized:

$$\text{GFR/BSA} \propto \frac{\text{UV creatine}}{\text{P creatinine} \times \text{BSA}} \propto \frac{\text{Height}}{\text{P creatinine}} .$$

In spite of the overstretched logic this formula works well (Schwartz *et al.*, 1976). The exact constant needed to predict GFR in ml min^{-1} per 1.73 m^2 will depend a little on the method of creatinine measurement. There is broad agreement, however, on the following formula (Counahan *et al.*, 1976; Davies *et al.*, 1982; Morris *et al.*, 1982):

$$\text{GFR ml min}^{-1} \text{ per } 1.73 \text{ m}^2 = \frac{\text{Height (cm)} \times 40}{\text{P creatinine } (\mu\text{mol l}^{-1})} .$$

The Schwartz formula is simple to apply. The rules are:

1. The formula only applies to somatically normal children of 3 years and older who are free from muscle disease.

2. In this age range a height/creatinine ratio of >2.16 predicts normal GFR with 95% probability.
3. An individual prediction of GFR by this method has a wide confidence limit except when renal function is reduced.
4. Repeated estimates in an individual patient give a clear indication of change of renal function. These estimates should be plotted in any child with a prospect of changing function, as illustrated in Figure 4.1 (page 22).

There is now no place for creatinine clearance in paediatric practice as the Schwartz formula gives superior results. The corollary is that the plasma creatinine in children of 3 years and above should only be interpreted in the knowledge of the child's height.

Plasma creatinine in infants
The use of plasma creatinine in younger patients is made more complex because of the rapidly changing GFR, and the Schwartz formula has not been adequately compared with standard methods. Nevertheless, some authors suggest that the principle still holds (Zacchello *et al.*, 1982). Pending definitive answers most nephrologists use the formula to observe the change of estimated GFR with time. Again by plotting the results and interpreting the graph in comparison with the physiological maturation (see Figure 5.1) one gets a better idea of the clinical course.

The plasma creatinine of the newborn, which reflects maternal creatinine and perhaps muscle damage occurring during labour, falls immediately after birth, depending on the infant's renal function, gestational age and the contraction of the extracellular water compartment in the adaptation to extrauterine life. In the first hours, therefore, the plasma creatinine alone is a weak indicator of renal function. In these circumstances the best guide is the table of normal ranges of plasma creatinine corrected for gestational maturity produced by Rudd *et al.* (1983) (Table 5.1).

Table 5.1 95% confidence limits of plasma creatinine in neonates

Gestation	Age (days)				
(weeks)	2	7	14	21	28
28	40–220	23–145	18–118	16–104	15–95
30	30–192	20–132	17–107	15–95	13–87
32	27–175	19–119	15–97	14–86	12–78
34	24–158	17–109	14–88	12–78	11–71
36	23–143	16–98	12–80	11–71	10–64
38	20–130	13–89	12–72	10–64	9–59
40	18–118	13–81	10–66	9–57	9–53

References

Chantler, C. and Barratt, T. M. (1972) Estimation of glomerular filtration rate from plasma clearance of 51-chromium edetic acid. *Archives of Disease in Childhood*, **47**, 613–617

Chantler, C., Garnett, E. S., Parsons, V. *et al.* (1969) Glomerular filtration rate measurement in man by the single injection method using ^{51}Cr-EDTA. *Clinical Science*, **37**, 169–180

Coultard, M. G. and Hey, E. N. (1984) Weight as the best standard for glomerular filtration in the newborn. *Archives of Disease in Childhood*, **59**, 373–375

Counahan, R., Chantler, C., Ghazali, S. *et al.* (1976) Estimation of glomerular filtration rate from plasma creatinine concentration in children. *Archives of Disease in Childhood*, **51**, 875 878

Davies, J. G., Taylor, C. M., White, R. H. R. *et al.* (1982) Clinical limitations of the estimation of glomerular filtration rate from height/plasma creatinine ratio: a comparison with simultaneous ^{51}Cr edetic acid slope clearance. *Archives of Disease in Childhood*, **57**, 607–610

Du Bois, D. and Du Bois, E. F. (1916) Clinical calorimetry. X. A formula to estimate the approximate surface area if the height and weight be known. *Archives of Internal Medicine*, **17**, 863–871

Griffiths, P. D., Drok, Z., Green, A. *et al.* (1988) Comparison of EDTA and DTPA slope clearances in children with reflux (submitted)

Haycock, G. B., Schwartz, G. J. and Wisotsky, D. H. (1978) Geometric method for measuring body surface area: a height–weight formula validated in infants, children, and adults. *Journal of Pediatrics*, **93**, 62–66

Kainer, G., McIlveen, B., Hoschl, R. *et al.* (1979) Assessment of individual renal function in children using ^{99m}Tc-DTPA. *Archives of Diseases in Childhood*, **54**, 931–936

McCrory, W. W. (1972) *Developmental Nephrology*, Harvard University Press, Cambridge, Mass., pp. 95–108

Morris, M. C., Allanby, C. W., Toseland, P. *et al.* (1982) Evaluation of a height/plasma creatinine formula in the measurement of glomerular filtration rate. *Archives of Disease in Childhood*, **57**, 611–615

Newman, E. V., Bordley, J. and Winternitz, J. (1944) The interrelationships of glomerular filtration rate (mannitol clearance), extracellular fluid volume, surface area of the body and plasma concentration of mannitol. A definition of extracellular fluid clearance determined by following the plasma concentration after a single injection of mannitol. *Bulletin of the John Hopkins Hospital*, **75**, 253–268

Piepsz, A., Denis, R., Ham, H. R. *et al.* (1978) A simple method for measuring separate glomerular filtration rate using a single injection of 99m Tc-DTPA and the scintillation camera. *Journal of Pediatrics*, **93**, 769–774

Rudd, P. T., Hughes, E. A., Placzek, M. M. *et al.* (1983) Reference ranges for plasma creatinine during the first month of life. *Archives of Disease in Childhood*, **58**, 212–215

Schwartz, G. J., Haycock, G. B., Edelmann, C. M. and Spitzer, A. (1976) A simple estimate of glomerular filtration rate in children derived from body length and plasma creatinine. *Pediatrics*, **58**, 259–263

White, R. H. R. and Taylor, C. M. (1984) The nonoperative management of primary vesicoureteric reflux. In *Management of Vesicoureteric Reflux* (ed. J. H. Johnston), Williams and Wilkins, Baltimore/London

Winterborn, M. H., Beetham, R. and White, R. H. R. (1977) Comparison of plasma disappearance and standard clearance techniques for measuring glomerular filtration rate in children with and without vesicoureteric reflux. *Clinical Nephrology*, **7**, 262–270

Zacchello, G., Bondio, M., Saia, O. S. *et al.* (1982) Simple estimate of creatinine clearance from plasma creatinine in neonates. *Archives of Disease in Childhood*, **57**, 297–300

Chapter 6

Urine concentration

Introduction

The ability to conserve body water is of paramount importance to all terrestrial animals, and this function is jeopardized by various renal diseases and both pituitary or nephrogenic diabetes insipidus. The capacity for urinary concentration depends on the osmolality of the renal medulla and the permeability of the collecting ducts to water; the latter being under the control of antidiuretic hormone (ADH).

In the proximal convoluted tubule 70% of the filtered salt and water is recovered, but there is a negligible osmolar gradient between the tubular lumen and the interstitium of the cortex. The loop of Henle runs into the medulla. In the ascending limb sodium is actively transported into the interstitium but water is unable to follow passively and so the sodium concentration in the medulla increases and dilute urine is delivered to the distal convoluted tubule (Figure 6.1). Urea is passively absorbed along with water both in the proximal tubule and in the collecting duct itself. The medullary solutes would be readily washed out by the peritubular blood were it not for the unique anatomy of the vasa recta which act as a counter-current exchange mechanism. These thin-walled blood vessels are supplied by the *efferent* arterioles of the juxta medullary nephrons and, like the loops of Henle, run a hairpin course towards the renal papillae. The plasma within them will already have an increased oncotic pressure as a fraction of the plasma water will have been filtered by the glomerular capillary bed leaving proteins in increased concentration. This blood is then able to equilibrate both with the increasing interstitial osmolality as it flows towards the tip of the papilla, and with the decreasing solute concentration on its return to the cortex. High blood flow through the vasa recta would have the effect of reducing the efficiency of the counter-current exchange and it has recently been shown that blood flow in these vessels is under the direct control of ADH (Zimmerhackl, Robertson and Jamison, 1985) and the renin angiotensin system (Faubert, Chou and Porush,

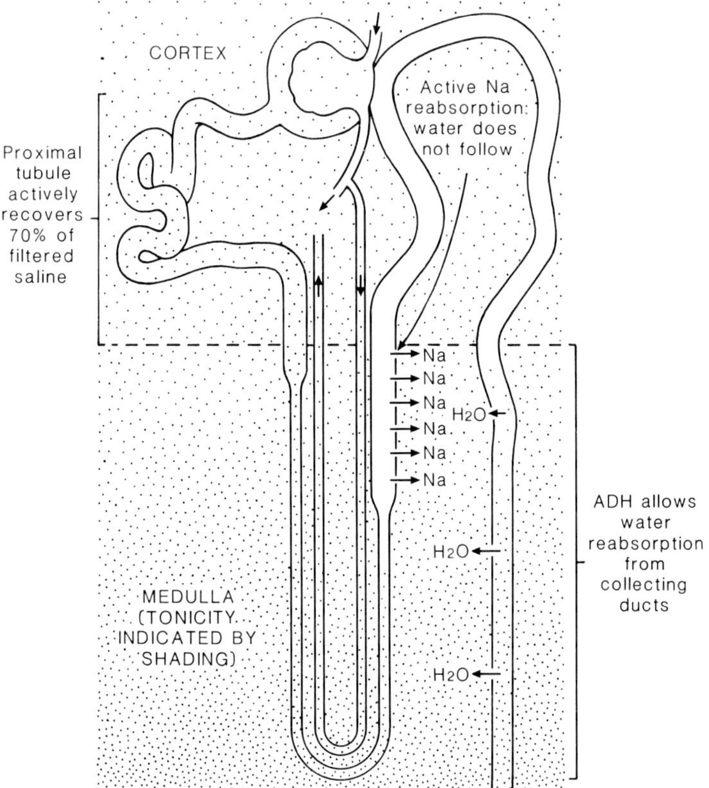

Figure 6.1 The counter-current exchange mechanism

1987). It should also be pointed out that the conventional explanation for the maintenance of medullary tonicity is incomplete
(Jamison, 1987).

The dilute fluid in the distal convoluted tubule drains into the
collecting ducts, which then traverse the hypertonic medulla to
emerge as the ducts of Bellini on the cribriform tip of the papilla.
Permeability of the collecting ducts and thus the passive absorption
of water depend on ADH and this hormone governs the final
concentration of the urine.

ADH secretion is regulated both by the hypothalamic osmorecep-
tors and by volume receptors in the great veins, the signal from
volume depletion having precedence.

At all ages the tonicity of the renal medulla is influenced by the
urea concentration and thus by the dietary protein intake. This

effect, however, has been shown to have a major influence on the maximal concentrating capacity in infants. When given very high solute feeds, even young infants are capable of achieving maximal urine osmolalities which are close to those found in adults (Edelmann, Barnett and Troupkou, 1960). However, in practical terms the concentration capacity in infancy is reduced (Polacek *et al.*, 1965), although the ability to excrete a water load is proportionately little different from that of adults. For this reason stressed neonates encounter greater problems with hydropenia than with water excess.

Concentration defects should be suspected in any infant with unexplained irritability, failure to thrive, fever, dehydration or hypernatraemia. Older children are more likely to present with nocturnal enuresis accompanied by a clear history of polyuria and polydipsia.

Tests of urinary concentration

The overnight fluid deprivation test
This test was carefully evaluated by Edelmann *et al.* in 1967. It is inappropriate to perform the investigation outside hospital in any child strongly suspected of having diabetes insipidus, as serious dehydration may occur. However, the test has the advantage that it can be performed at home by other cooperative subjects and normal data have been produced for children above 2 years of age. It is worth pointing out that patients resent this investigation only marginally less than a formal water deprivation study, and it is not unknown for them to cheat!

The child has a normal midday meal, but drinks are prohibited from noon. A 'dry' supper is given, i.e. fluid-containing foods such as jelly, ice cream or gravy are avoided. On retiring to bed the child voids and discards the urine. Thereafter urine is saved. On rising in the morning the child voids into a container, after which normal eating and drinking can be resumed. The osmolality of the collected urine is measured by the method of depression of freezing point. The mean for the test in both sexes and throughout the age range 2–16 years is 1089 mosmol kg^{-1} with a working range of normal from 873 to 1305 mosmol kg^{-1}.

The DDAVP test
DDAVP (desmopressin) is a synthetic analogue of ADH which on a molecular basis has approximately five times the antidiuretic effect, but only a small fraction of the vasoconstrictor properties of the natural hormone. After a single dose it has a duration of action of up

to 12 hours and because it is well absorbed across the nasal mucosa it can be administered without injection.

No special preparation is needed but it is a wise precaution to weigh the child as a baseline measurement at the start of the test and to record fluid intake and urine output. If the patient has compulsive water drinking it is theoretically possible to induce water intoxication if input continues while output is blocked. By contrast to impose water restriction if the child truly has nephrogenic diabetes insipidus may result in dehydration. In infants their usual fluid intake is halved for the two feeds after giving DDAVP.

The older child is asked to clear the nose by blowing, and not to sniff or sneeze while the DDAVP is given. The dose chosen is estimated to provide maximal antidiuretic effect; 40 µg in adults, 20 µg in children, 10 µg in infants. The drops are instilled into the nostrils and the head rotated from side to side to disperse the DDAVP over a wide area of mucosa. One hour later the child is asked to void and this urine is discarded. Thereafter urine is collected, preferably as separate aliquots from the period 1–3 hours and 3–5 hours after administration. The osmolality achieved in normals is not as high as that found in prolonged water restriction. However, a usable range of values has been produced (Monnens *et al.*, 1981); the mean for children of more than 1 year is 991 mosmol kg^{-1} and the lower limit of normal 800 mosmol kg^{-1}. Normal infants are able to achieve an osmolality of 600 mosmol kg^{-1} by 6 months.

This is a well-tolerated and trouble-free test. Patients with pituitary diabetes insipidus will usually achieve concentrations close to the normal range (completely normal with regular DDAVP dosage), whereas those with renal disorders will show impairment. However, on a single occasion this test will not demonstrate subtle impairment of concentration capacity in renal parenchymal disease. By repeating the test during the course of an illness the change in an individual can be observed more reliably. For example, in the 4–6 months after acute renal parenchymal infection it is possible to see a rise of some 200 mosmol kg^{-1} in the concentration capacity determined by this test. However, both figures may fall within the envelope of normal range. Children with nephrogenic diabetes insipidus are readily discerned as, in the absence of hypernatraemia, they rarely have a urine osmolality in excess of 300 mosmol kg^{-1}.

Formal water deprivation study
Whereas children with normal renal function can be expected to achieve a maximum urine concentration in a uniform time period, this is not so for patients with reduced concentration capacity. The

end-point of this test is not time but loss of 3% of body weight, at which point it is assumed that there is a maximal stimulus to urinary concentration.

The patient is examined to ensure that hydration is normal to start with. The *body weight is accurately recorded* and a target weight of 3% below this is set. Fluids are withheld, although dry foods are permitted. The body weight, and in infants heart rate and blood pressure, are monitored. The child is encouraged to void at regular intervals (infants may require catheterization) and urine is collected for osmolality. This is a miserable test for the child and it is a kindness to report the osmolality immediately so that if a reading is obtained in excess of 870 mosmol kg^{-1} (600 mosmol kg^{-1} in infants) the test can be stopped. This result could be accepted as an adequate indication of normality for most clinical decisions. At 3% dehydration both plasma and urine osmolalities are measured. The former confirms the stimulus to water conservation, the latter is the maximal concentrating capacity.

Summary

- The DDAVP test is the simplest and safest way of identifying a *renal* concentrating defect.
- In pituitary diabetes insipidus it is necessary to show a concentrating defect in the absence of DDAVP; use the overnight fluid deprivation test.
- In infants particularly weigh the child and monitor for dehydration in any water deprivation test.

References

Edelmann, C. M., Barnett, H. L., Bricks, H. and Soriano, J. (1967) A standardized test of renal concentrating capacity in children. *American Journal of Disease in Children*, **114**, 639–644

Edelmann, C. M., Barnett, H. L. and Troupkou, V. (1960) Renal concentrating mechanism in newborn infants, effect of dietary protein and water content, role of urea and responsiveness to anti diuretic hormone. *Journal of Clinical Investigation*, **39**, 1062–1069

Faubert, P. F., Chou, S.-Y. and Porush, J. G. (1987) Regulation of papillary plasma flow by angiotensin II. *Kidney International*, **32**, 472–478

Jamison, R. J. (1987) The renal concentrating mechanism. *Kidney International*, **32**, suppl. 21, S43–50

Monnens, L., Smulders, Y., van Lier, H. and de Boo, T. (1981) DDAVP test for assessment of renal concentrating capacity in infants and children. *Nephron*, **29**, 151–154

Polacek, E., Vocel, J., Neugebauerova, L., Sebkova, M. and Vechetova, E. (1965) The osmotic concentrating ability in healthy infants and children. *Archives of Disease in Childhood*, **40**, 291–295

Zimmerhackl, B., Robertson, C. R. and Jamison, R. L. (1985) Effect of arginine vasopressin on renal medullary blood flow. A video microscopic study in the rat. *Journal of Clinical Investigation*, **76**, 770–778

Chapter 7

Tubular function

Hydrogen ion

Hydrogen ion homeostasis is of major importance to biochemical and physiological functions. By far the greatest contribution to the excretion of acid is the respiratory loss of carbon dioxide and thus carbonic acid. An adult excretes 13 000 mmol carbonic acid day^{-1} via the lungs whereas an anephric patient may require only 100 mmol day^{-1} of bicarbonate to maintain normal hydrogen ion (H^+) balance.

Normal renal tubular cells can excrete H^+ against a gradient to achieve a minimum urine pH of less than 5.0 (free acid). Moreover the secreted H^+ ions combine with a variety of buffers present in the filtrate, the most important of these being phosphate. This allows a greater quantity of H^+ to be excreted, the buffer-bound H^+ being measurable as titratable acid. Hydrogen ion is also carried as the ammonium (NH_4^+) ion. The tubular cells hydrolyse glutamine to ammonia (NH_3), which readily diffuses into the filtrate where it combines with H^+. Ammonia production by the kidney is increased in acidaemia and this helps to regulate acid excretion. The total acid excretion is therefore the sum of free hydrogen ion, titratable acid and ammonium iron. If there is any bicarbonate leakage this would need to be deducted from the total to give the net balance of acid excreted:

$$\text{net acid excretion} = H^+ + \text{titratable acid} + NH_4^+ - HCO_3^-.$$

Plasma bicarbonate is freely filtered at the glomerulus and more than 85% is reabsorbed in the proximal tubules. In proximal tubular diseases the reabsorptive process may fail and bicarbonate is lost in the urine. As the plasma bicarbonate falls and acidosis develops, less bicarbonate is presented to the glomerulus, filtration is reduced and so a smaller load is presented to the tubules. A new steady state may then be reached which is within the tubules' capacity, albeit subnormal, for bicarbonate recovery. The distal H^+ secretory mechanism continues to function and urinary pH may fall below 5.5. A reduced maximal tubular reabsorption of bicarbonate occurs in isolation as renal tubular acidosis (RTA) type II (see below).

Metabolic acidosis

Metabolic acidosis comes about either by a primary reduction of plasma bicarbonate (renal or enteric bicarbonate loss) or by hydrogen ion excess (failed H^+ excretion or an excess H^+ load). Figure 7.1 illustrates a scheme for pursuing this in clinical practice. The normal range of venous plasma chloride and bicarbonate is 95–108 mmol l^{-1} and 22–26 mmol l^{-1} respectively. One should remember that bicarbonate is not usually directly measured but estimated from the pH and PCO_2 of the sample. The anion gap is calculated as follows:

$$\text{anion gap} = (Na^+ + K^+) - (Cl^- + HCO_3^-).$$

Normally this is between 14 mmol l^{-1} and 20 mmol l^{-1}. If either bicarbonate wasting or failed hydrogen ion excretion causes acidosis, the plasma chloride rises and the anion gap remains unchanged. However, if the primary problem is an accumulation of other acids (e.g. organic acids) the gap is usually greater than 25 mmol l^{-1}.

In patients with hyperchloraemic metabolic acidosis measurement of urinary pH, which needs to be checked with a hydrogen ion

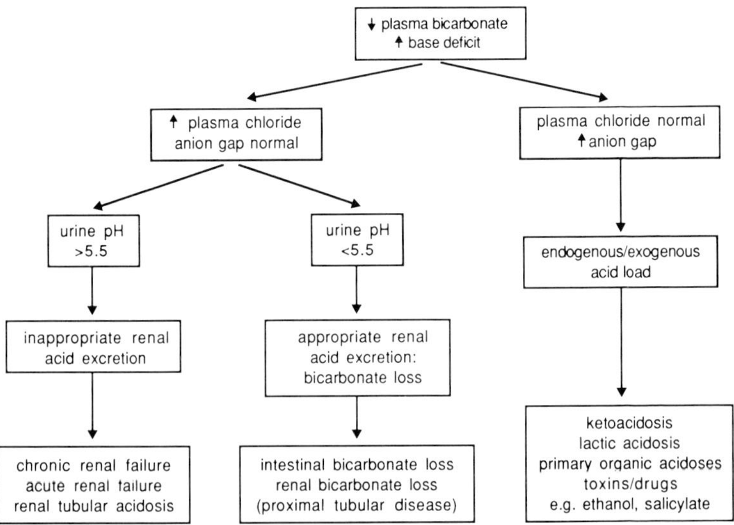

Figure 7.1 A simplified scheme for investigating metabolic acidosis

electrode, helps to indicate whether tubular secretion of H^+ is appropriate.

In normal children the reduction in urinary pH which occurs as a response to increasing metabolic acidosis follows the graph shown in Figure 7.2. From this it can be seen that if the acidosis is sufficient to depress the plasma bicarbonate to $< 20\,\text{mmol}\,l^{-1}$ a urinary pH < 5.2 would be an appropriate response whereas a urine pH > 5.5 is good evidence of a renal acidification defect. If the latter, the defect may be secondary either to structural renal damage and chronic renal failure or due to renal tubular acidosis (RTA). Renal imaging and an estimate of GFR will determine which. With regard to the former investigation it should be noted that in any form of RTA nephrocalcinosis may occur. This is because in acidaemia calcium is mobilized from bone and there is both hypercalciuria and hypocitraturia, the combined effect of which is to reduce calcium solubility in the tubular fluid and promote crystal formation.

If the child has anatomically normal kidneys (nephrocalcinosis excepted) and normal GFR this indicates RTA but does not itself determine which subtype. However, given the plasma bicarbonate and urinary pH criteria above, proximal tubular bicarbonate wasting type II RTA is effectively excluded.

If in the initial presentation of acidosis a plasma bicarbonate concentration of $< 20\,\text{mmol}\,l^{-1}$ was not observed, further acidosis can be induced with oral ammonium chloride. There is no universal dosage but the range of $2.5\text{--}5.5\,\text{mmol}\,\text{kg}^{-1}$ body weight will induce a mild to moderate acidaemia in normals. It is a nauseating solution which can be disguised in a flavoured drink and given in small frequent aliquots. Ammonium chloride should not be given to patients with hepatic dysfunction. Once the plasma bicarbonate has reached $< 20\,\text{mmol}\,l^{-1}$ the above criteria can be applied.

Often the most practical next step is to treat the patient with oral

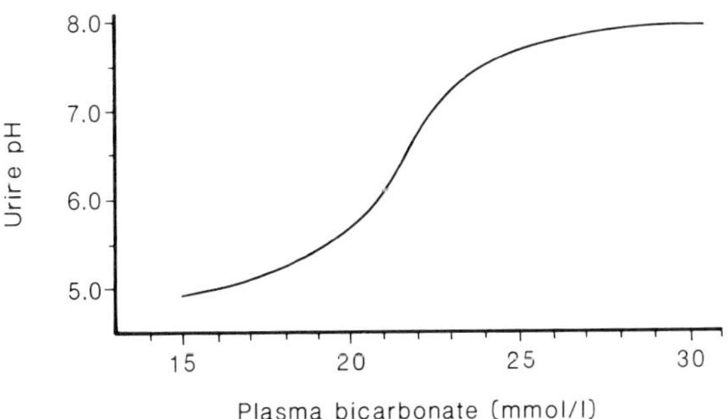

Figure 7.2 The physiological response of urinary pH to systemic acidaemia

sodium bicarbonate at a dose of 3–5 mmol kg^{-1} body weight day^{-1}. This will fully correct distal RTA but would be insufficient to balance a bicarbonate wasting disorder; children with type II RTA usually require doses of 10–15 mmol day^{-1}.

Another simple way of determining whether renal tubular acidosis is proximal or distal is to measure the PCO_2 in simultaneously collected capillary blood and urine once the urine has been made maximally alkaline (pH > 7.8) by bicarbonate loading (Donckerwolke *et al.*, 1983). In distal RTA there is an inability to increase urinary PCO_2. Neither sample must be exposed to the air as the PCO_2 will rapidly fall and it is therefore important to seal the capillary tube used for the blood sample, and preferable to collect the urine via a fine catheter into a syringe, which is immediately capped. The laboratory should be advised in advance of this test so that samples can be processed without delay. A difference between urine and blood PCO_2 of < 2.0 kPa (15 mmHg) indicates distal and > 2.7 kPa (20 mmHg) proximal RTA.

Alternatively confirmation of proximal tubular bicarbonate loss can be obtained with a bicarbonate titration study. In this the child must have a very low plasma bicarbonate to start with, and this is increased steadily by an intravenous bicarbonate infusion. The plasma bicarbonate concentration at which the urinary pH exceeds 6.8 (the level above which urine is assumed to contain bicarbonate) is taken as the threshold. In normal children this is between 22 mmol l^{-1} and 26 mmol l^{-1}.

Probably the most common RTA observed in childhood, and one which accompanies structural renal diseases such as dysplasia or reflux nephropathy, consists of a mixture of both distal and proximal features (type III RTA). In these patients or others in whom the above screening procedures give inconclusive results, further information can be gained with both the ammonium chloride load test (Edelmann *et al.*, 1967; Monnens, 1974) and the assessment of bicarbonate reabsorption (Soriano, Boichis and Edelmann, 1967). With these studies, which involve bladder catheterization and timed urine collections, the individual components of the equation for net acid excretion are determined at various degrees of acid–base disturbance. A full explanation of normal data is contained in these references.

Type IV RTA refers to a group of conditions in which there is failure of the normal mineralocortical response by the distal nephron. Aldosterone normally increases the activity of the cationic exchange in the distal tubule in which Na$^+$ is actively reabsorbed in exchange for K$^+$ and H$^+$. Failure of this system gives rise to acidosis, hyperkalaemia and salt wasting. The clinical features of the syndrome are exaggerated in neonates who are physiologically more dependent on distal tubular sodium recovery than are adults. Causes include various forms of the adrenogenital syndrome, hypoaldosteronism and pseudohypoaldosteronism.

Metabolic alkalosis

In metabolic alkalosis the plasma bicarbonate is elevated and compensatory hypoventilation leads to a rise in plasma carbon dioxide. The commonest cause for this in childhood is an enteric, selective chloride loss; a good example being that which occurs in pyloric stenosis. The urine will be practically chloride free and chloride replacement will quickly re-establish normal acid–base homeostasis. Chronic alkali ingestion, a common cause for alkalosis in adults, is rare in childhood and would be quickly identified from the history.

In distinction from the above, an important cause of metabolic alkalosis, so-called 'chloride unresponsive' alkalosis, is seen when the tubule receives an inappropriate signal to excrete hydrogen ion. In all cases the urinary chloride excretion is increased. In the distal nephron aldosterone controls the cationic exchange mechanism in which sodium is recovered and potassium and hydrogen ion excreted. Any disorder enhancing the renin/angiotensin/aldosterone pathway, or any primary mineralocorticoid excess occurring, for example in Cushing's syndrome or more rarely in congenital adrenal hyperplasia or primary hyperaldosteronism, may induce this condition. This is in effect the opposite of type IV RTA. Just as hydrogen ion is excreted to excess so is potassium and the alkalosis is typically associated with hypokalaemia. Bartter's syndrome of hypokalaemic alkalosis, in which other tubular disturbances occur, usually presents with marked salt wasting and contraction of the extracellular fluid space, and is therefore unlike mineralocorticoid excess.

Measurements of tubular reabsorption/excretion

The clearance of any substance which is filtered by the glomerulus and then reabsorbed to some extent by the tubule can be compared with the clearance of inulin or more easily creatinine, which is similarly filtered but not handled by the tubules (Figure 7.3). In such a comparison time and body surface area cancel out so that the fractional excretion (FE) is as follows:

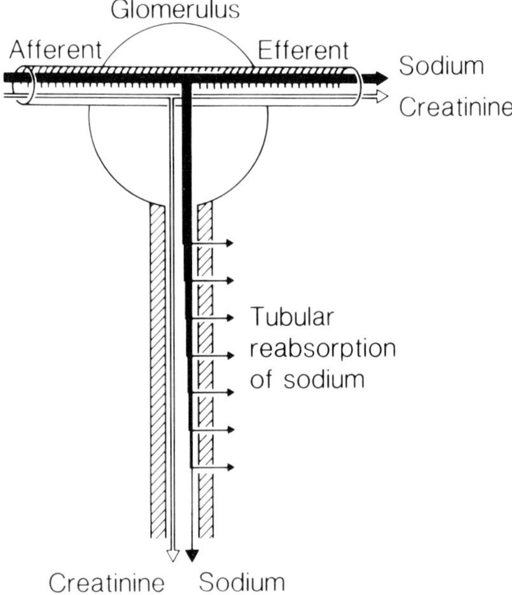

Figure 7.3 The concept of fractional excretion

$$\text{FE of } x = \frac{\text{clearance } x}{\text{clearance creatinine}} = \frac{Ux \times U \text{ creatinine}}{Px \times P \text{ creatinine}}.$$

That part of the filtrate which is reabsorbed is now

$1 - \text{FE of } x.$

This concept is useful in discerning some aspects of tubular function, especially where the plasma concentration of the test substance is maintained in a narrow range. The reabsorption of a compound may, however, vary depending on the rate at which it is delivered to the tubule and therefore on the plasma concentration. Conventional ways to express this are either to define the maximum rate of tubular transport ($Tm\ x$) or the threshold plasma concentration beyond which the substance is detectable in the urine. These concepts are relatively easy to apply and are useful in exploring both specific and generalized disturbances of tubular function.

In Fanconi's syndrome of generalized failure of proximal tubular reabsorption, sodium, bicarbonate, phosphate, glucose and amino acid recovery is reduced. Moreover reabsorptive processes in the distal nephron are swamped and mineralocorticoid-stimulated cation exchange is increased so that hypokalaemia is an important feature. In childhood the commonest cause of Fanconi's syndrome is the lysosomal storage disorder cystinosis.

Sodium

The quantity of sodium (Na) filtered and recovered each day is more than three times that contained in the whole of the extracellular fluid volume. More than 99% is reabsorbed, 85% of it in the proximal tubules. Failure to recover sodium is life threatening and it is therefore a good design point that sudden tubular incapacity is accompanied by a steep reduction in GFR and oliguric renal failure (Thurau and Boylan, 1976). In health the FE Na is well below 1% except in the newborn and preterm infant in whom this is approximately 2% and 5% respectively. An FE Na above these guidelines is pathological in a patient who is judged to be sodium depleted by signs of dehydration or weight loss, with or without hyponatraemia, and suggests that renal salt loss is the cause of the problem. In patients who have sustained surgical shock but whose renal adaptation is appropriate the FE Na will indicate avid sodium recovery (pre-renal failure). By contrast once hypoxic tubular damage has occurred the FE Na rises and this observation may have some limited clinical value (Mathew *et al.*, 1980; Pru and Kjellstrand, 1984).

Potassium

Potassium (K) is extensively recovered in the proximal tubule and in the ascending limb of the loop of Henle. In the distal nephron K is actively secreted so that FE K may well exceed unity during kaliuresis. A rise in plasma K is a powerful stimulus to aldosterone secretion and this has a role in the regulation of K homeostasis (Himathongham, Dluhy and Williams, 1975).

Calcium and magnesium

Plasma calcium (Ca) and magnesium (Mg) are partially bound to plasma proteins and form complexes with other ions. Only about half of the total plasma Ca is in the ionized form Ca^{2+}. Calcium is reabsorbed in the proximal tubule and changes in its absorption tend to mirror those of Na. Volume contraction by chronic administration of a thiazide diuretic, for example, will cause increased Ca reabsorption, part of the rationale for thiazide use in hypercalciuria and urolithiasis.

Marked changes in urinary Ca and Mg excretion are simply

judged against the normal range of urinary Ca/creatinine and Mg/creatinine ratios (Ghazali and Barratt, 1974). The normal upper limit for calcium/creatinine is 0.74 mmol mmol^{-1} and magnesium/creatinine 1.94 mmol mmol^{-1} (0.26 mg mg^{-1} and 0.41 mg mg^{-1} respectively).

Phosphate

Inorganic phosphate is freely filtered in the glomerulus and extensively reabsorbed in the proximal tubules. Plasma phosphate concentrations are higher in infancy and childhood than in adult life and the concentration depends largely on the rate of tubular recovery, the transport maximum for phosphate (Tm PO_4). Overall girls tend to have a higher excretion than boys of a similar age. The Tm PO_4, which is itself GFR dependent, is higher in childhood than in adult life (Kruse, Kracht and Gopfert, 1982) and is under hormonal control. Parathyroid hormone, and to a lesser extent calcitonin and oestrogens, have a phosphaturic effect, whereas vitamin D metabolites oppose this. A reduced reabsorption of phosphate is a major component of the generalized proximal tubular disturbance of Fanconi's syndrome.

In normal children the fractional excretion of phosphate has a very wide range of between 2% and 19% of the filtered load, and is therefore of limited clinical use. However, if the plasma phosphate and the fractional excretion are known, the term Tm PO_4/GFR, which is the most soundly based description of tubular phosphate handling, can be predicted using the nomogram of Walton and Bijvoet (1975) (Figure 7.4). Normal data for children of 6 years and older are given by Kruse, Kracht and Gopfert (1982) and for infants of less than 6 months by Bistarakis *et al.* (1986).

Glucose

The renal plasma threshold for glucose in normals is approximately 10 mmol l^{-1} (180 mg dl^{-1}) and the transport maximum is lower in preterm and normal infants (Brodehl, 1978a). Glucose recovery occurs extensively in the proximal tubule, and in health the amount excreted in the urine of adults has been shown to be approximately 200 μmol min^{-1} per 1.73 m^2, which gives urinary concentrations below the level detectable by most glucose oxidase reagent strips. Glycosuria detected by conventional urine analysis and occurring at a normal range of blood glucose is therefore an indication of reduced renal threshold. This occurs either as an isolated finding, in which case it is a consistent and benign feature (primary renal

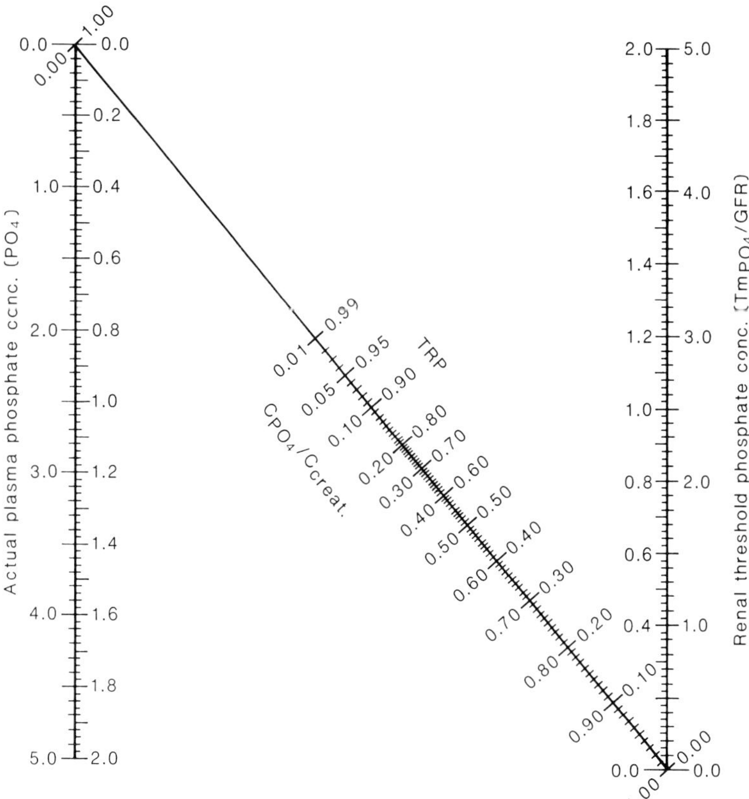

Figure 7.4 Nomogram for predicting the transport maximum for phosphate/GFR

glycosuria), or as part of Fanconi's syndrome or chronic renal failure from a wide variety of parenchymal diseases.

Amino acids

Plasma amino acids are filtered at the glomerulus and more than 90% of the filtered load is reabsorbed by the proximal tubule. Newborn infants have a generalized, mild aminoaciduria which represents a maturational process within the tubule. Hyperexcretion of amino acids can occur either because the plasma concentration is sufficiently elevated to overload normal tubular reabsorption ('overflow' aminoaciduria), as in phenylketonuria, or because of defects in tubular recovery ('renal' aminoaciduria). In the latter, there may be a generalized loss of amino acids, such as in Fanconi's syndrome from whatever primary cause, or specific patterns of aminoaciduria depending on the transport process involved.

Four main transport mechanisms have been described, and defects in each reported. Cystinuria, an autosomal recessive disorder which predisposes to cystine urolithiasis, is the commonest and an example of defective transport of dibasic amino acids. Lysine, arginine and ornithine are also excreted in excess. Disturbances of other transport systems include the iminoglycine, dicarboxylic and monocarboxylic/monoamine (Hartnup disease) groups. The subject has been well reviewed by Brodehl (1978b).

Most laboratories rely on chromatography to identify amino acids and gain semiquantitative information about each amino acid component. Experience is needed with this technique both to standardize for variations in urine creatinine concentration, and to compare the result with normal children of similar age. Chromatography should be performed in parallel on serum taken at the same time as the urine sample so as to distinguish between 'overflow' and 'renal' aminoaciduria. Always notify the laboratory of all drugs that the child is taking as some of them appear in the chromatogram and need to be distinguished.

References

Hydrogen ion
Donckerwolke, R. A., Valk, C., van-Wijngaargen-Peterman, M. J. *et al.* (1983) The diagnostic value of the urine to blood carbon dioxide tension gradient for the assessment of distal tubular hydrogen secretion in pediatric patients with renal tubular disorders. *Clinical Nephrology*, **19**, 254–258

Edelmann, C. M., Boichis, H., Soriano, R. J. and Stark, H. (1967) The renal response to acute ammonium chloride acidosis. *Pediatric Research*, **1**, 452–460

Monnens, L. (1974) A modification of the short ammonium chloride loading test in children. *Nephron*, **12**, 129–132

Soriano, J. R., Boichis, H. and Edelmann, C. M. (1967) Bicarbonate reabsorption and hydrogen ion excretion in children with renal tubular acidosis. *Journal of Pediatrics*, **71**, 802–813

Measurements of tubular reabsorption/excretion
Bistarakis, L., Voskaki, I., Lambadaridis, J. *et al.* (1986) Renal handling of phosphate in the first six months of life. *Archives of Disease in Childhood*, **61**, 677–681

Brodehl, J. (1978a) Renal glycosuria. In *Pediatric Renal Disease* (ed. C. M. Edelmann), Little, Brown and Co., Boston, pp. 1036–1046

Brodehl, J. (1978b) Renal hyperaminaciduria. In *Pediatric Diseases of the Kidney* (ed. C. M. Edelmann), Little, Brown and Co., Boston

Ghazali, S. and Barratt, T. M. (1974) Urinary excretion of calcium and magnesium in children. *Archives of Disease in Childhood*, **49**, 97–101

Himathongham, T., Dluhy, R. and Williams, G. H. (1975) Potassium, aldosterone, renin interrelationship. *Journal of Clinical Endocrinology and Metabolism*, **41**, 153–

Kruse, K., Kracht, U. and Gopfert, G. (1982) Renal threshold phosphate concentration (Tm PO_4/GFR). *Archives of Disease in Childhood*, **57**, 217–223

Mathew, O. P., Jones, A. S., James, E. *et al.* (1980) Neonatal renal failure: usefulness of diagnostic indices. *Pediatrics*, **65**, 57–60

Pru, C. and Kjellstrand, C. M. (1984) The FE_{Na} test is of no prognostic value in acute renal failure. *Nephron*, **36**, 20–23

Thurau, K. and Boylan, J. W. (1976) Acute renal success. The unexpected logic of oliguria in acute renal failure. *American Journal of Medicine*, **61**, 308–315

Walton, R. J. and Bijvoet, O. L. M. (1975) Nomogram for derivation of renal threshold phosphate concentration. *Lancet*, **ii**, 309–310

Chapter 8

Imaging: plain films

Radiation hazards

Although nearly all patients in the paediatric age-group will not be pregnant it is prudent to remember that this may not always be the case. Until recently a guideline known as 'the 10-day rule' was in operation in all X-ray departments. This rule stated that an examination of the abdomen of a female of reproductive capacity which involved the use of ionizing radiation should be confined to the first 10 days of the menstrual cycle. In this way only the unfertilized ovum would be irradiated.

Recent advice from the National Radiological Protection Board (1985) supersedes these earlier recommendations. Its comments are based on a document published by the International Commission on Radiological Protection (ICRP, 1984) which states: 'During the first ten days following the onset of a menstrual period there can be no risk to any conceptus, since no conception will have occurred. The risk to a child who had previously been irradiated *in utero* during the remainder of a four week period following the onset of menstruation is likely to be so small that there need be no special limitation on exposures required within these four weeks.' Organogenesis does not occur until after formation of the 'primitive streak' at about 15 or 16 days post fertilization. The only dividing cells during the first 4 weeks following the first day of the last menstrual period are those that line the extra-embryonic coelomic cavity, damage to which will not result in malformation of any liveborn child (Pochin, 1986). Thus, we now have, in effect, a '28-day rule'.

Chromosomal damage may result from irradiation of the early conceptus but the vast majority of such cases will spontaneously abort at an early stage. Leukaemia and central nervous system malignancies may follow later exposure *in utero* and develop during the first decade. Mental retardation may also be induced by the absorption of small doses of radiation (Otake and Schull, 1984).

It behoves all clinical staff requesting the irradiation of their patients to determine whether they could be pregnant and to confine such investigations to the 28-day period following the first day of the last menstrual cycle unless clinical circumstances override such considerations.

The plain abdominal radiograph

This is a simple investigation which can yield much useful information. The renal area may be shown to better advantage if the exposure is made following a large drink (Smith, 1987). The distended stomach then displaces other bowel gas away from the underlying kidneys. Caudad angulation of 30° of the X-ray beam, either alone or in combination with a distended stomach, will also improve visualization of the renal areas by projecting colonic contents below the kidneys. Items for study on the plain film are:

1. Renal outlines
2. Other soft-tissue shadows, e.g. size of the bladder
3. Calcification and calculi
4. Gas in the urinary tract
5. Skeleton.

Renal outlines

Renal outlines are defined by virtue of the presence of the perirenal fat. It should be remembered that the loss of a renal outline on plain films is not necessarily associated with non-visualization of that kidney during excretion urography. Causes of loss of renal outline are listed in Table 8.1.

Renal size
Large or small; unilateral or bilateral. This is better assessed by excretion urography and is discussed more fully in Chapter 9.

Renal position
In the normal position the left kidney lies a little higher than the right and the long axes of both kidneys lie parallel to the psoas outlines, i.e. with the lower poles further from the midline (Figure 8.1). It is quite uncommon to see an ectopic kidney on plain films; this entity is more usually evident by non-visualization of a kidney in its orthotopic position. The most common congenital abnormality of position to be diagnosed on the plain film is the horseshoe kidney (Figure 8.2). In this condition the long axis of each kidney is more vertical than usual, being parallel to the spine rather than parallel to

Table 8.1   Loss of renal outline on the plain abdominal radiograph

1. Technical factors	Poor radiography, overlying bowel shadows
2. Congenital absence	1:1000 live births
	Increased incidence of extrarenal abnormalities (ventricular septal defect, meningomyelocoele, oesophageal atresia, tracheo-oesophageal fistula, imperforate anus and skeletal anomalies)
	The solitary normal kidney will show compensatory hypertrophy
3. Post-nephrectomy	Residual perinephric fat preserves an apparent renal outline
	There may be evidence of surgical resection of the 12th rib
4. Displaced or ectopic	Presacral, crossed ectopia or intrathoracic kidney
5. Perinephric haematoma	+/− other signs of trauma, e.g. fractured ribs
	Scoliosis concave to the injured side
6. Perinephric abscess	Scoliosis concave to the affected side
	+/− localized ileus or gas in the perinephric space
7. Tumour	When perinephric fat is replaced by tumour

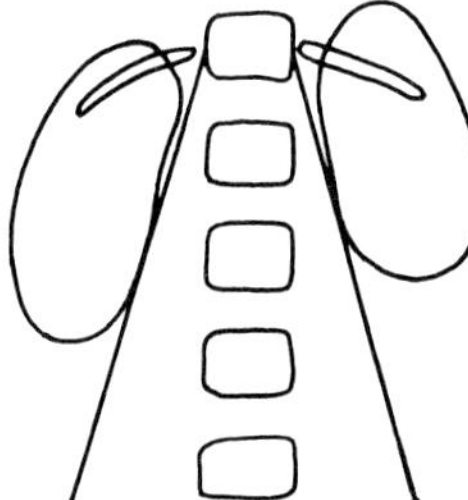

Figure 8.1 Normal position of the kidneys with their long axes parallel to the outline of the psoas muscles

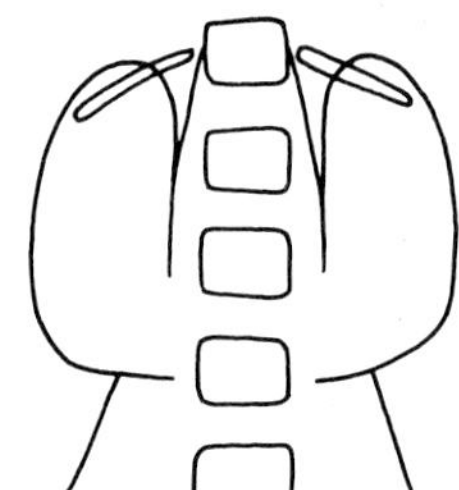

Figure 8.2 A horseshoe kidney with the long axis of each renal mass parallel to the spine; the medial outline of each lower pole is lost because of the isthmus

the outline of the psoas muscles. In addition the medial edge of each lower pole cannot be defined because renal isthmus replaces perirenal fat. A kidney may be displaced by an adjacent mass, e.g. adrenal haemorrhage or neuroblastoma.

Renal shape

Subtle alterations of renal shape are not to be diagnosed on the plain film. Massive enlargement, such as occurs in polycystic disease, and focal enlargement due to Wilm's tumour may be evident by virtue of displacement of bowel shadows.

Bladder size

When the plain film is requested as the only investigation it is useful to expose the film after micturition. Further information will then be obtained about bladder size following voiding.

Calcification

There are a number of causes of calcifications in the urinary tract:

1. Calculi – renal, ureteric or bladder
2. Nephrocalcinosis
3. Dystrophic calcification in diseased tissue.

To be certain that calcification or calculus is truly renal it must be shown to be constantly related to the kidney. This can be done in one of several ways:

1. Comparison of radiographs exposed during inspiration and expiration (Figure 8.3).
2. Comparison of straight and oblique views of the kidney.
3. Tomography. This is a radiographic technique in which an exposure is made while the X-ray tube and film move in opposite directions relative to a fixed pivot point. Structures in the patient at the same level as the fulcrum remain in focus while those either side of that level are blurred out.

It should be remembered that an underlying abnormality of the urinary tract can place a urinary tract density in an unusual location.

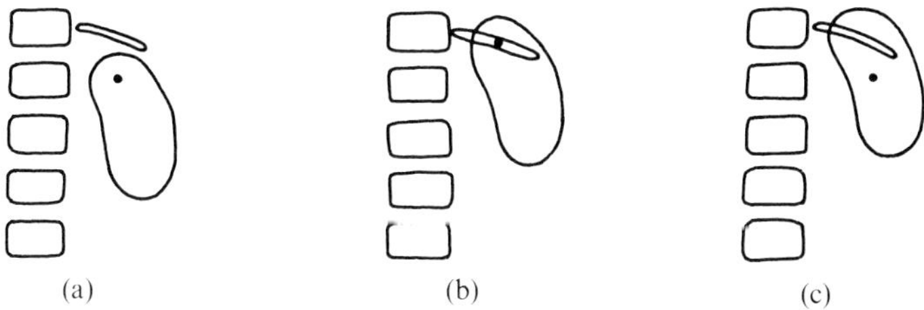

(a) (b) (c)

Figure 8.3 Inspiration and expiration films to determine if a density is related to a kidney. (a) A density overlies a renal outline on the routine film exposed during inspiration. (b) A film exposed at full expiration shows the density to have maintained a constant relationship to the kidney and so it must lie within the kidney. (c) When the density does not maintain a constant relationship to the kidney it cannot be within it

For example, a calculus in a markedly dilated renal pelvis or ectopic kidney may lie outside of the expected renal area.

Calculi
Three patterns of incidence can be recognized (Barratt and Ghazali, 1977):

1. Infection – particularly with *Proteus* species. These calculi are composed of organic matrix and magnesium ammonium phosphate and are predominantly found in the upper tracts. Infection may be associated with stasis, i.e. the situation in the obstructed or atonic system. One-third of children in this group have an underlying urological abnormality other than vesico-ureteric reflux (VUR).
2. Metabolic disorders – cystinuria, hyperoxaluria, xanthinuria, etc.
3. Diet – the predominant cause in Turkey and the Far East and possibly related to a diet of cereals and rice. Stones occur, predominantly in the bladder, and are composed of ammonium acid urate and oxalate.

Several factors should be considered when evaluating a possible urinary tract calculus (Elkin, 1983).

DENSITY

The radiographic density of the calculus may suggest the chemical composition. Opaque calculi contain calcium salts (calcium phosphate/calcium oxalate, calcium oxalate, calcium phosphate or calcium phosphate/magnesium ammonium phosphate). Calcium oxalate stones are more radiopaque than triple phosphate stones. Poorly opaque calculi are likely to be cystine (due to cystinuria) and the non-opaque calculi, which of course will not be seen on the plain abdominal radiograph, are composed of uric acid or xanthine. Calculi are usually homogeneously dense but sloughed papillae, in papillary necrosis, are radiolucent with a rim of calcification peripherally and bladder calculi may have a lamellated appearance.

SHAPE

This may be distinctive, e.g. the staghorn calculus of the renal pelvis, the stallate bladder calculus or the triangular sloughed papilla of papillary necrosis.

MOBILITY

A calculus in an undilated calyx will remain in a fixed position whereas a calculus in a dilated calyx or pelvis will move freely within the containing viscus. Bladder calculi will be mobile within the bladder shadow and this is best demonstrated by comparison of supine and prone or supine and erect films.

POSITION AND NUMBER

Eighty per cent of calculi in a recent series (Breatnach and Smith, 1983) were located in the kidneys: 24% of their children had multiple calculi and in 18% calculi were bilateral. This stresses the need to look for more than one stone.

COMPARISON WITH PREVIOUS RADIOGRAPHS

An opacity within the line of a ureter, and which has previously been shown to be in the renal area, may be confidently diagnosed as a renal calculus.

Nephrocalcinosis

This is parenchymal calcification and may be either medullary or cortical in location (Figure 8.4). Nephrocalcinosis may be associated with nephrolithiasis.

MEDULLARY (PYRAMIDAL)

1. Renal tubular acidosis. Nephrocalcinosis occurs almost always with a distal tubular defect because it is here that there is loss of calcium in the urine. Nephrocalcinosis is rare in proximal renal tubular acidosis.
2. Hyperparathyroidism, most often primary. There may be other signs in the skeleton (see below).
3. Hypercalciuria, secondary to steroid therapy, Cushing's disease or idiopathic.
4. Oxaluria. This may be the result of a primary disorder of glyoxalate metabolism or there may be an enteric hyperoxaluria due to increased absorption of oxalate secondary to Crohn's disease or distal small bowel resection. The kidneys may be diffusely dense.
5. Wilson's disease.

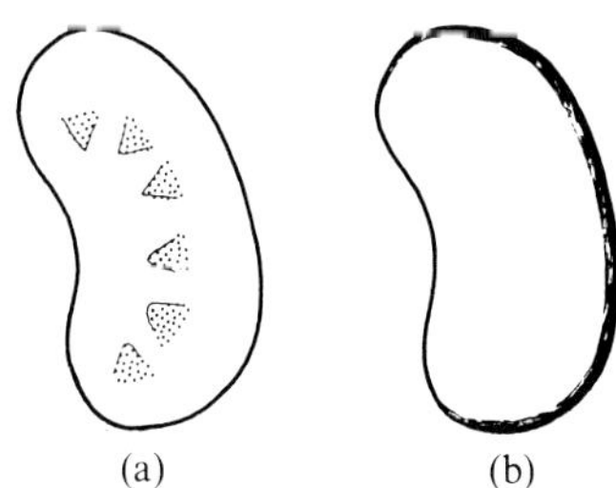

Figure 8.4 Nephrocalcinosis. (a) Medullary, within the renal papillae. (b) Cortical

CORTICAL

1. Acute cortical necrosis. Classically tramline calcification but which is usually not seen until several weeks after the onset of renal failure.
2. Chronic transplant rejection.
3. Chronic glomerulonephritis. Rare.

Dystrophic calcification in diseased tissue
This is usually in one kidney only or in part of one kidney. Causes to be considered include:

1. Wilms' tumour. Dystrophic calcification occurs in less than 10% of cases and there is usually a plainly visible, soft-tissue renal mass. Calcifications are scattered throughout the tumour but may be difficult to see on the routine plain film if there are overlying gas and faeces. The lateral projection may be useful in such circumstances. In patients under the age of 1 year the benign tumour, mesoblastic nephroma, presents an identical picture.
2. Tuberculosis. Calcification has a variable appearance but is typically multifocal with calcification elsewhere in the urinary tract.
3. Xanthogranulomatous pyelonephritis. Calcifications in this condition are mostly calculi which originally produced the obstruction which became secondarily infected and resulted in tissue destruction. Dystrophic calcification can, however, occur in the damaged tissue, In children the disease is commonly focal but may, rarely, be diffuse.

Gas in the urinary tract

This is suggested by gas shadows which conform to the position and shape of the pelvicalyceal systems, ureters or bladder. In the neonatal period the commonest cause is a recto-vesical fistula in association with a high-type imperforate anus. In the older child consideration should be given to ureters which have been diverted into the colon and a fistula due to Crohn's disease.

Skeleton

Important information may be obtained from a study of the skeleton, both on the abdominal radiograph and by review of other sites, particularly the hand and wrist.

The spine
There may be evidence of widening of the spinal canal. The interpedicular distance on the anteroposterior view of the abdomen

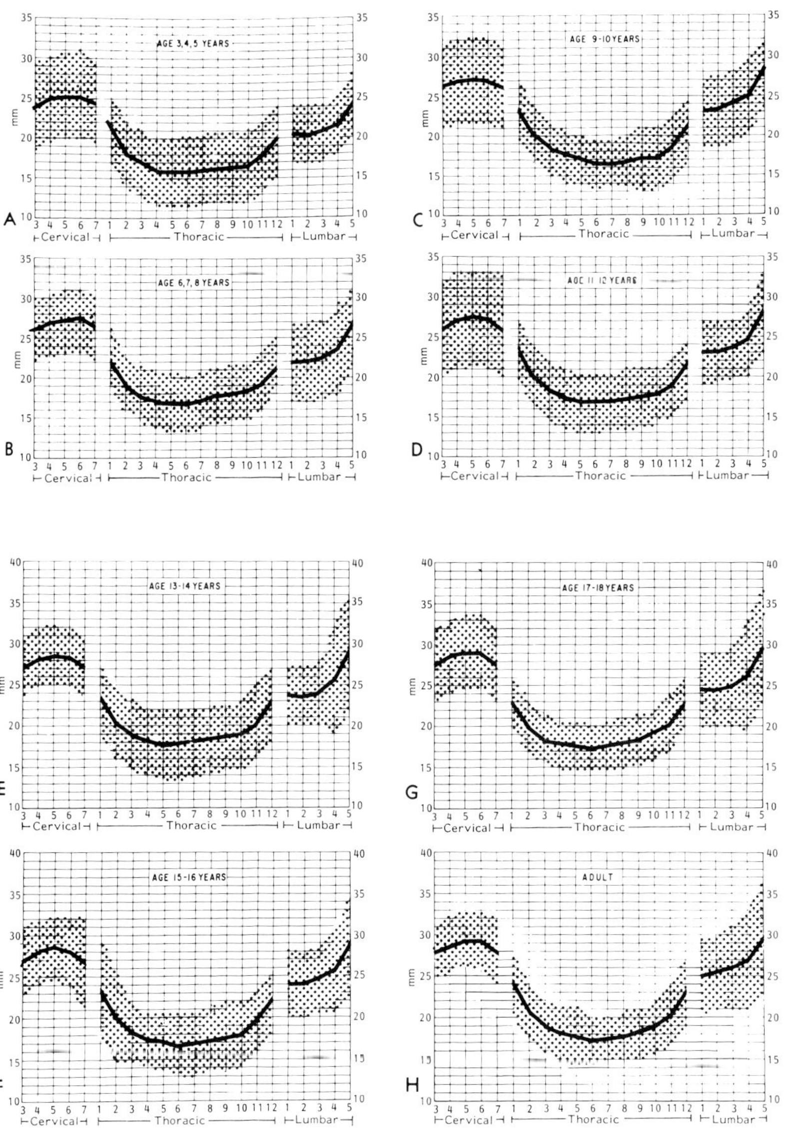

Figure 8.5 Normal interpedicular distances. Mean and upper and lower limits for differing ages. (From Hinck, Clark and Hopkins, 1966, by kind permission of the authors and publishers. © American Roentgen Ray Society, 1966)

Table 8.2   Causes of excessive widening of the lumbosacral interpedicular distances

1.	Meningomyelocoele	Fusiform distribution of widened inter-pedicular distances Disc spaces are narrowed and vertebral bodies appear widened Spinous processes and laminae are absent. Scoliosis in 50–70% of cases
2.	Diastematomyelia	The spur is bony, and therefore visible radiologically, in 33% Fifty per cent of cases occur between L1 and L3. Widening of interpedicular distances is common but not necessarily at the same level as the spur
3.	Intraspinal mass	Usually a shorter history than the above two

normally increases in the lumbosacral region. By reference to charts of age-related normal measurements (Figure 8.5) excessive widening may be determined. In such cases a short differential diagnosis must be considered (Table 8.2).

A disturbance of micturition in association with widening of the spinal canal is an indication for myelography.

Spina bifida occulta, i.e. fusion defects of the laminae and spinous processes of L5, S1 and/or S2, often in association with skin and soft-tissue abnormalities, is to be found in approximately 20% of the population. Progressive closure of defects occurs with maturation and many regard the finding as a normal variant. However, Galloway and Tainsh (1985) and others have shown a higher incidence of bony defects in patients with lower urinary tract dysfunction.

The pelvis
The pelvis should be examined for signs of rickets or hyperparathyroidism. Diastasis of the symphysis pubis accompanies ectopia vesicae and hypospadias (see Figure 9.3).

Rickets and osteomalacia

The characteristic changes of rickets are identified at the metaphyses and growth plates prior to closure while osteomalacia is seen in mature bone. Since both result from the same pathophysiological mechanisms, findings representative of rickets and osteomalacia may be present in individuals affected just prior to growth plate fusion. However, for the sake of convenience, each condition is described separately.

Radiological diagnosis of rickets

Rickets will be most obvious in regions of active growth. Thus in order of decreasing sensitivity the sites of highest radiographic yield will be the costochondral junctions, distal femur, proximal humerus, both ends of tibia and the distal radius and ulna (Park, 1932). In the adolescent the iliac crest apophyses show the changes best.

The changes at the growth plate reflect the disordered increase in cell growth and deficient mineralization of osteoid in the zone of provisional calcification on the metaphyseal side of the growth plate. The following constitute the characteristic radiographic changes (Pitt, 1981) (Figure 8.6).

1. Generalized non-specific osteopenia.
2. Axial widening of the growth plate, which represents the earliest specific sign.
3. A decrease in density of the zone of provisional calcification follows. (The zone of provisional calcification is the normal dense line on the metaphyseal side of the growth plate.)
4. Further widening of the growth plate occurs as the disease progresses and the zone of provisional calcification becomes irregular.
5. Fraying and flaring of the metaphysis are due to accumulation of uncalcified osteoid at the metaphysis.
6. As the amount of uncalcified osteoid accumulates abnormal stresses are placed on the more central areas of the metaphysis and cupping occurs.
7. A thin bony spur may extend from the margin of the metaphysis to surround the uncalcified growth plate.

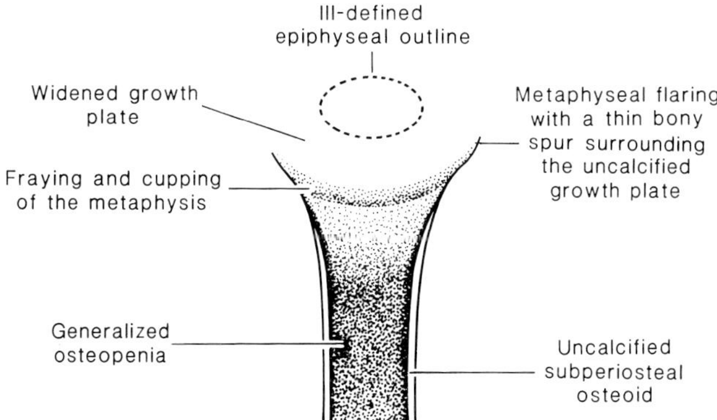

Figure 8.6 Diagrammatic representation of the radiological changes of rickets

8. Uncalcified osteoid beneath the periosteum gives the appearance of a periosteal reaction.
9. The margin of the epiphysis is analogous to the provisional zone of calcification and thus the changes at the epiphysis are those of deossification and blurring at its periphery.
10. Stresses applied to softened bones result in bowing deformities of long bones.

The signs of rickets may be masked by systemic malnutrition when there is also deficient production of osteoid.

Radiological diagnosis of osteomalacia
The predominant radiological manifestation is osteopenia, a non-specific sign which does not facilitate the easy diagnosis of osteomalacia. Secondary bone trabeculae are lost resulting in the residual primary trabeculae appearing more prominent and bone has a coarsened look. Unlike osteoporosis the residual trabeculae have blurred margins because they are coated with poorly calcified osteoid. Looser's zones or pseudofractures are characteristic of osteomalacia and may precede other radiographic changes (Steinbach and Noetzli, 1964). They appear as lucencies with sclerotic margins orientated at right angles to the cortex and extending incompletely across the bone (Figure 8.7). They are commonly symmetrical and typical sites are the ribs, axillary margins of the scapula, superior and inferior pubic rami, inner margins of the

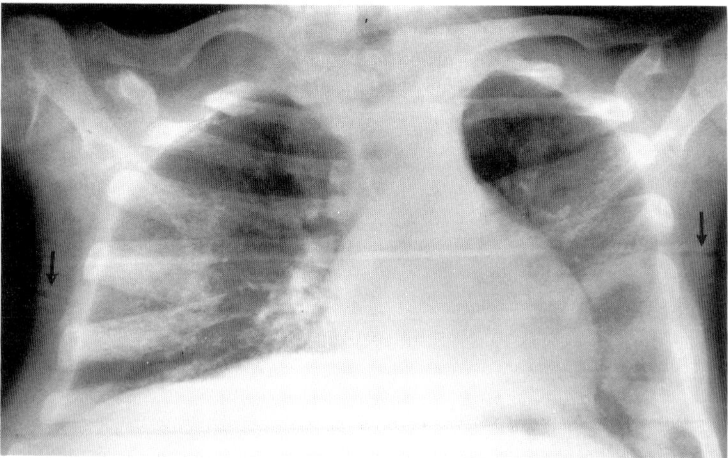

Figure 8.7 Bilaterally symmetrical Looser's zones (*arrow*) on the lateral aspects of both scapulae

proximal femora and posterior margins of the proximal ulnae. True fractures may occur through these areas of weakening.

Renal bone disease

The skeletal changes of chronic renal disease may comprise:

1. Rickets/osteomalacia
2. Osteitis fibrosa (hyperparathyroid bone disease)
3. Osteosclerosis
4. Osteopenia
5. Extraskeletal calcification.

Renal glomerular failure may exhibit all of the above features, collectively known as renal osteodystrophy. The radiological picture in renal tubular failure is that of rickets or osteomalacia.

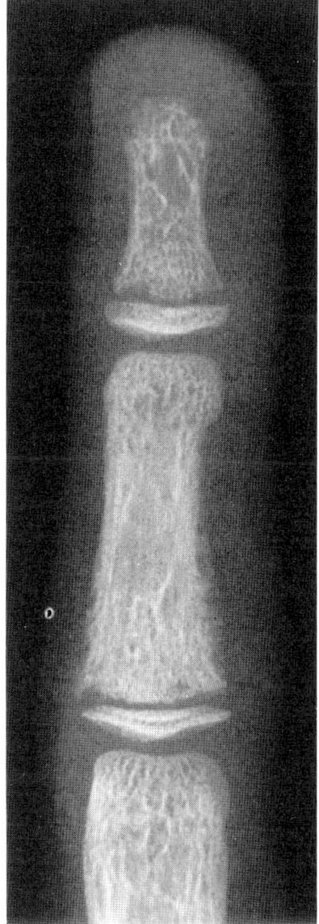

Figure 8.8 Subperiosteal bone resorption in hyperparathyroidism produces a lace-like outline to the cortical bone. The changes are most marked in the middle phalanx

Renal glomerular failure – renal osteodystrophy
The radiological changes reflect the secondary hyperparathyroidism and deficiency of $1,25(OH)_2D$. The major abnormalities are osteitis fibrosa cystica (hyperparathyroid bone disease), rickets or osteomalacia (or both), osteosclerosis and osteopenia. Rickets is usually the presenting feature in children although the changes of hyperparathyroidism may be quite prominent (Pitt, 1981). The earliest sign of the latter is subperiosteal resorption of bone on the radial side of the middle phalanx of the middle finger, which appears radiologically as a lace-like outline of the cortex (Figure 8.8). With more advanced disease all of the phalanges show this sign, there is resorption of distal phalangeal tufts and subperiosteal resorption on the medial sides of the femoral necks and proximal tibiae. Resorption of bone at the femoral necks may be so severe that the appearance has been likened to a rotting fence post. Slipped upper femoral epiphysis (Figure 8.9) may occur and has been recorded in 10% of children with chronic renal disease (Mehls *et al.*, 1975). The slip may, initially, be clinically silent and three radiographic signs which may precede slipping and alert the clinician are bilateral subperiosteal erosion on the medial aspect of the femoral neck, widening of the growth plate and coxa vara (Goldman, Lane and Salvati, 1978). Subperiosteal resorption at joint margins, e.g. the

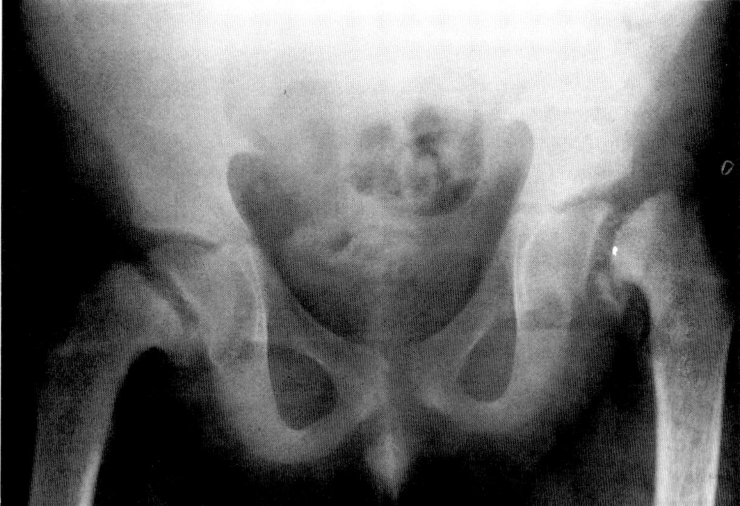

Figure 8.9 Slipped upper femoral epiphyses. The epiphyseal growth plates are wide on both sides and both capital epiphyses have slipped, the slip being more severe on the left side

acromioclavicular and sacroiliac joints and symphysis pubis, produces widening of those joints.

Areas of increased density (osteosclerosis) are due to excessive accumulation of osteoid. Although per unit volume osteoid is deficient in mineral it presents as increased density because of the increased volume of osteoid present. Characteristic sites for osteosclerosis are in the superior and inferior end plates of the spine (the 'rugger jersey' spine; Figure 8.10) and the metaphyses of long bones (Figure 8.11).

Osteopenia, i.e. decreased bone density, is accompanied by cortical thinning and is due to a combination of rickets/osteomalacia and hyperparathyroidism. Steroid therapy, possibly following renal transplantation, will accentuate the loss of bone density. Fractures may occur.

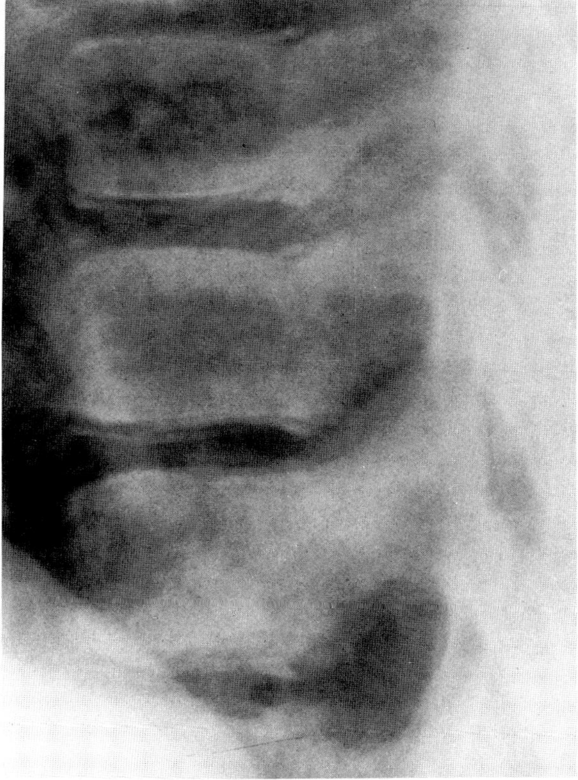

Figure 8.10 Rugger-jersey spine

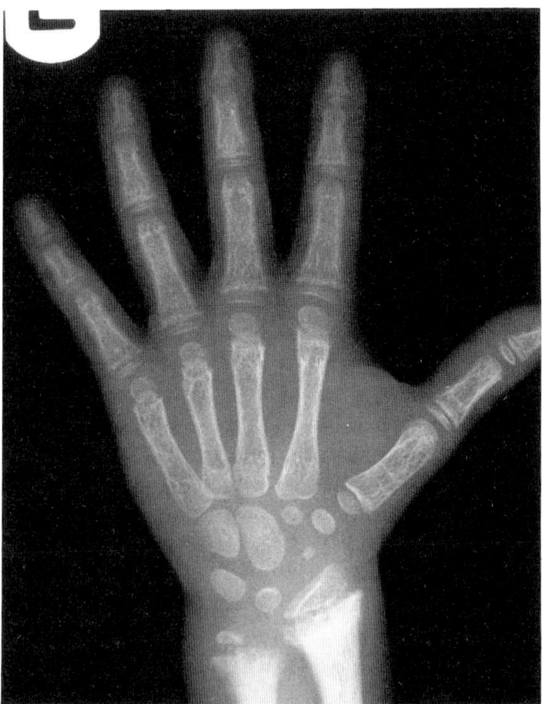

Figure 8.11 Renal osteodystrophy. There are radiological changes of rickets, secondary hyperparathyroidism and bone sclerosis. This latter feature is particularly evident in the radial and ulnar metaphyses

Soft-tissue calcification may occur in the kidneys, lungs, skin, arteries and periarticular areas.

Musculoskeletal abnormalities following dialysis and transplantation

Although many of the musculoskeletal manifestations in children treated with haemodialysis, peritoneal dialysis or renal transplantation are due to renal osteodystrophy, some of these manifestations are modified during treatment and additional manifestations may be encountered that relate to the specific mode of therapy (Resnick and Niwayama, 1981). Thus a limited skeletal survey should be carried out at the commencement of treatment to act as a baseline for comparison with future radiological examinations. Adequate hae-

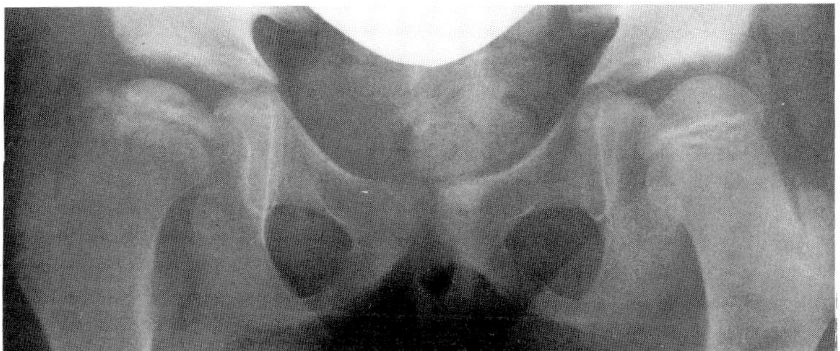

Figure 8.12 Avascular necrosis of the right femoral capital epiphysis

modialysis will result in the resolution of the bone changes of renal osteodystrophy but poorly managed patients suffer increasing osteopenia and spontaneous fractures, most commonly of the ribs (Simpson *et al.*, 1971). Soft-tissue and arterial calcification are frequent in patients on haemodialysis. Soft-tissue calcification may regress during dialysis but arterial calcification is usually progressive. Infective complications are well-recognized complications of haemodialysis and are predisposed to by the use of arteriovenous shunts, corticosteroids and immunosuppressive agents in patients who already have impaired host resistance.

Avascular necrosis of bone is a well-known complication following transplantation. Steroid administration is the most likely cause although this complication does occur in patients who have not received steroids. The most common site of ischaemic necrosis following renal transplantation is the femoral head. The earliest radiological sign is a linear subchondral lucency which represents a subarticular fracture. Later fragmentation, collapse, sclerosis and cyst formation are seen, the articular space being preserved (Figure 8.12).

Occasionally small cystic lesions are seen in the hands and wrists of patients undergoing chronic haemodialysis (Resnick and Niwayama, 1981).

References and further reading

Radiation hazards
International Commission on Radiological Protection (1984) Statement from the 1983 Washington meeting of ICRP. *Annals of ICRP*, **14**, no. 1
National Radiological Protection Board (1985) *ASP8*, HMSO, London.
Otake, M. and Schull, V. J. (1984) In utero exposure to A bomb radiation and mental retardation: a reassessment. *British Journal of Radiology*, **57**, 409–414

Pochin, E. E. (1986) Annotation. The 10-day recommendation. *Clinical Radiology*, **37,** 105–106

The plain abdominal radiograph

Barratt, T. M. and Ghazali, S. (1977) The aetiology of renal stones in children. In *Paediatric Implications for some Adult Disorders. Report of the Fourth Unigate Paediatric Workshop* (ed. D. Barltrop), Fellowship of Postgraduate Medicine, London, pp. 35–40

Breatnach, E. and Smith, S. E. W. (1983) The radiology of renal stones in children. *Clinical Radiology*, **34,** 59–64

Elkin, M. (1983) Calcification in the urinary tract. In *Plain Film Approach to Abdominal Calcifications* (eds S. R. Baker and M. Elkin), W. B. Saunders, Philadelphia, pp. 39–46

Galloway, N. T. M. and Tainsh, J. (1985) Minor defects in the sacrum and neurogenic bladder dysfunction. *British Journal of Urology*, **57,** 154–155

Hinck, V. C., Clark, W. M. Jr and Hopkins, C. E. (1966) Normal interpediculate distances (minimum and maximum) in children and adults. *American Journal of Roentgenology*, **97,** 141–153

Smith, S. E. W. (1987) Management of urinary tract infection. *Archives of Disease in Childhood*, **62,** 978

Rickets and osteomalacia

Park, E. A. (1932) The Blackader lecture on some aspects of rickets. *Canadian Medical Association Journal*, **26,** 3

Pitt, M. J. (1981) Rickets and osteomalacia. In *Diagnosis of Bone and Joint Disorders* (eds D. Resnick and G. Niwayama), W. B. Saunders, Philadelphia, pp. 1802–1859

Steinbach, H. L. and Noetzli, M. (1964) Roentgen appearance of the skeleton in osteomalacia and rickets. *American Journal of Roentgenology*, **91,** 955–972

Renal bone disease

Goldman, A. B., Lane, J. M. and Salvati, E. (1978) Slipped capital femoral epiphyses complicating renal osteodystrophy. *Radiology*, **126,** 333–339

Grech, P., Martin, T. J., Barrington, N. A. and Ell, P. J. (1985) Renal bone disease. In *Diagnosis of Metabolic Bone Disease*, Chapman and Hall Medical, London, pp. 131–157

Mehls, O., Ritz, E., Krempien, B. *et al.* (1975) Slipped epiphyses in renal osteodystrophy. *Archives of Disease in Childhood*, **50,** 545–554

Pitt, M. J. (1981) Rickets and osteomalacia. In *Diagnosis of Bone and Joint Disorders* (eds D. Resnick and G. Niwayama), W. B. Saunders, Philadelphia, pp. 1682–1720

Musculoskeletal abnormalities following dialysis and transplantation

Resnick, D. and Niwayama, G. (1981) Parathyroid disorders and renal osteodystrophy. In *Diagnosis of Bone and Joint Disorders*, W. B. Saunders, Philadelphia, pp. 1802–1859

Simpson, W., Kerr, D. N. S., Hill, A. V. L. and Siddiqui, J. Y. (1971) Skeletal changes in patients on regular haemodialysis. *Radiology*, **107,** 313–320

Chapter 9

Imaging: contrast radiology

Excretion urography

Excretion urography (EU) is the most complete method of examining the child's urinary tract because it gives excellent information about structure and, to a lesser degree, function. In complex cases it is often *the* investigation which gives the overall perspective. It does, however, suffer a number of disadvantages:

1. Radiation dose.
2. Morbidity, and rarely mortality, of contrast medium administration.
3. Venepuncture.
4. Poor results when renal function is poor, i.e. the newborn and those in renal failure.

As a primary screening tool it is rapidly being replaced by ultrasonography (US) with or without nuclear medicine imaging.

Indications

1. Abnormal or equivocal renal US. Excretion urography will show the functional element of the ultrasound abnormality and clarify the US findings.
2. Signs and symptoms suggestive of a ureteric calculus. Ultrasonography will demonstrate the ureteric dilatation produced by the calculus but may fail to show the cause.
3. Trauma, when there is an isolated renal injury. The majority of injuries are managed conservatively and EU is necessary to confirm the presence of a normal contralateral kidney. When trauma to other intra-abdominal viscera is suspected computerized tomography with contrast medium enhancement is preferable.

Contraindications

1. Pregnancy – see Chapter 8.
2. A previous severe adverse reaction to contrast medium. This carries a 30% risk of a similar reaction on a subsequent occasion so consideration must be given to a different imaging modality such as US or nuclear medicine, which may be able to answer the clinical question. If EU is definitely required a low osmolar contrast medium (LOCM) should be used in preference to conventional high osmolar contrast media (see below) and pre-medication with prednisolone 12 and 4 hours prior to the investigation may also be beneficial.
3. Acute urinary tract infection. This may produce secondary upper tract dilatation, the significance of which will be difficult to interpret. In the acute situation US should be used to exclude a surgical condition such as a pyonephrosis due to obstruction and further investigation should wait until at least 4 weeks after the infection has been treated.

Contrast medium

Intravascular contrast media are water-soluble, iodine-containing compounds. With the exception of iodamide, which is handled by both glomerular filtration and tubular secretion, all other media are excreted by glomerular filtration only. The administration of conventional intravascular contrast media, which are ionic salts of tri-iodinated benzoic acid derivatives, may produce a number of adverse effects mediated via differing mechanisms:

Effects due to hypersensitivity
1. Allergic: urticaria, sneezing, conjunctivitis, rhinitis, broncho-spasm, angioneurotic oedema.
2. Acute anaphylaxis: in a previously sensitized individual.
3. Anaphylactoid reactions: in a non-sensitized individual.

Anaphylaxis may be initiated with or without complement activation and contrast media also have a direct histamine-releasing effect on mast cells, basophils and platelets.

Effects due to chemotoxicity
1. Direct effects on red cell morphology.
2. Contrast media are weakly protein bound and the degree of protein binding correlates with inhibition of the enzyme acetyl cholinesterase, the effects of which include vasodilatation, brady-cardia, hypotension, bronchospasm and urticaria. There is also a

cholinergic link between chemoreceptor trigger zone in the brain and the emesis centre. Among the new LOCM, ioxaglate (Hexabrix) has the greatest propensity to induce vomiting and also has a greater effect on acetyl cholinesterase inhibition than other contrast media (Manhire, Dawson and Dennet, 1984).
3. Iodine itself may be directly responsible for enzyme inhibition and other aspects of chemotoxicity.

Hyperosmolarity effects
Conventional ionic contrast media are hypertonic, with osmolarities of 1200–2000 mosmol kg^{-1} water, i.e. 4–7 times the osmolarity of blood. The administration of a hyperosmolar load into a young child will have adverse effects on:

1. Haemodynamics
2. Cardiac function
3. Endothelium
4. Erythrocyte deformability.

The new generation of LOCM have osmolarities of approximately one-third that of conventional agents and are indicated for paediatric use because they have been shown to reduce the incidence of all types of adverse side-effects (Spataro, 1984). They are, however, more expensive than conventional agents and financial stringencies may restrict their use to those who will derive particular benefit (Grainger, 1984):

1. Babies and young infants.
2. Children who have had a previous severe allergic reaction to contrast medium or who have a strong allergic history.
3. Children with impaired renal or cardiac function.
4. Diabetics. Diabetes predisposes to contrast medium-induced nephrotoxicity but LOCM are less nephrotoxic (Dawson, 1985).
5. Children with sickle cell anaemia (Rao *et al.*, 1982).

Intravascular contrast medium should not be given in the absence of resuscitation equipment, emergency drugs and a hospital resuscitation team.

Dosage
Using a contrast medium containing approximately 400 mg iodine ml^{-1} (Conray 420, Niopam 370, Omnipaque 350, Ultravist 370) 1 ml kg^{-1} up to 50 ml gives satisfactory results. When renal function is impaired the volume will need to be increased to 2 ml kg^{-1}. Contrast media in common usage are listed in Table 9.1.
The injection is given intravenously over at least 1 min to limit

Table 9.1   Intravascular contrast media in common usage

Proprietary name	*Chemical name of anion*	*Manufacturer*
Conventional high osmolarity contrast media		
Conray	Iothalamate	May & Baker
Hypaque	Diatrizoate	Sterling
Urografin	Diatrizoate	Schering
Uromiro	Iodamide	E. Merck
Low osmolarity contrast media		
Hexabrix	Ioxaglate	May & Baker
Niopam	Iopamidol	E. Merck
Omnipaque	Iohexol	Nycomed
Ultravist	Iopromide	Schering

intercompartmental fluid shifts. Occasionally, because of technical difficulties with venepuncture, only a few millilitres of contrast medium may be injected. It is usually worth while taking a radiograph at this point rather than repeating the venepuncture because an adequate urogram may be obtained. The previous practice of giving a subcutaneous injection of contrast medium mixed with hyaluronidase to those infants with poor venous access is no longer acceptable and these children should either be imaged with US or radionuclides or be referred to an institution where venepuncture may be more successful.

Patient preparation

1. Oral laxative, e.g. senna, will decrease the amount of bowel contents which would otherwise obscure the renal images.
2. The need for dehydration to improve the density of renal opacification is debated but is probably not necessary. Abstinence from solid food for 4 h to reduce the risk from vomiting induced by the contrast medium is, however, recommended. Infants, those in renal failure and very ill children should not be dehydrated and in these cases the investigation may be scheduled prior to a feed.
3. Investigation of a diabetic child should be carried out at the start of the day with the morning dose of insulin and breakfast being omitted. A mild degree of hyperglycaemia may be tolerated for a short period and insulin and food can be given at the conclusion of the investigation.

Films

A plain radiograph, using a low kilovoltage, which includes the renal areas and bladder before the administration of contrast medium is essential to:

1. Exclude subtle calcification and small calculi which would be missed following contrast medium injection. Oblique views, films in expiration and inspiration or tomography may be employed at this stage to confirm the presence of calcification (see Chapter 8).
2. Exclude prohibitive factors such as excessive faecal loading of the bowel or residual contrast medium, particularly barium, from a previous radiological examination.
3. Make final adjustments to exposure factors.

The exact sequence of films following contrast medium injection will vary between departments and be tailored to the particular clinical problem but a typical sequence would be:

1. Immediate film of the renal areas – this shows the nephrogram, i.e. the renal parenchyma opacified by contrast medium in the renal tubules. It is the most useful film for studying the renal outlines. The density of the nephrogram is related to the plasma concentration of contrast medium and glomerular filtration rate so a poor nephrogram may be improved by a further injection of contrast medium.
2. Five-minute film of the renal areas – taken with 30° caudad angulation of the tube to throw the faecal-laden transverse colon clear of the kidneys. By 5 min contrast medium has begun to opacify the calyces and pelvis.
3. Ten-minute film of the entire urinary tract.
4. Twenty-five minute film of the entire urinary tract.

Supplementary films and techniques may be indicated in certain situations:

1. Tomography – when overlying bowel obscures the renal outlines.
2. Renal window view (Hope and Campoy, 1955). When excessive bowel gas interferes with satisfactory visualization of the kidneys a carbonated beverage will produce a gas-filled stomach which acts as a window through which the kidneys can be seen.
3. Prone abdomen – may demonstrate drainage of contrast medium from the pelvis and may also provide better visualization of the ureters.
4. After-micturition film. The principal value of this film is to demonstrate a return to normal of dilated upper tracts with the

relief of bladder pressure, to assess bladder emptying, to aid the diagnosis of bladder tumours and, uncommonly, to demonstrate a urethral diverticulum in females (Gerber and Brown, 1985).

5. *Delayed films* – may be necessary for up to 24 h in cases of obstructive uropathy and in the neonatal period because of diminished renal function.

6. *Films following a diuretic or water load* – to clarify a possible pelvi-ureteric junction obstruction. When a diuresis is provoked, the dilated, but unobstructed upper tract will empty of opacified urine but the obstructed upper tract will dilate further.

Complications

Complications are almost entirely due to the administration of contrast medium and have been discussed above. They may also be classified in terms of severity:

1. Trivial reactions: those that do not interfere with the examination and require only firm reassurance, e.g. urticaria, flushing.

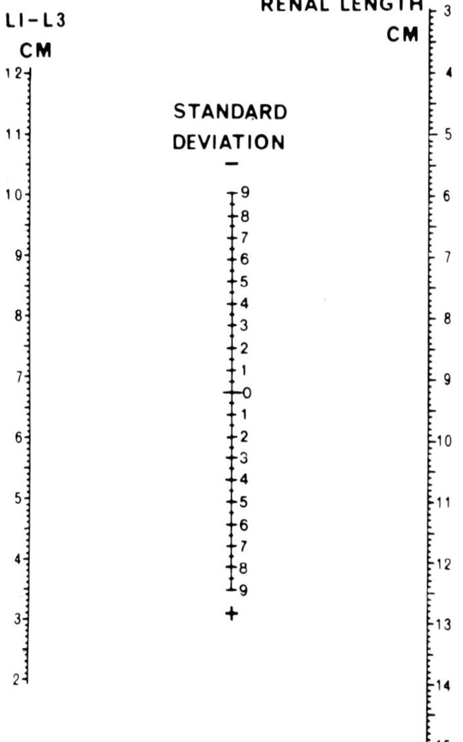

Figure 9.1 Nomogram for assessing renal length in standard deviations by reference to the L1–L3 distance (From Eklöf and Ringertz, 1976a, by kind permission of the authors and publishers)

2. Minor reactions: those that interfere with the examination but do not require treatment, e.g. vomiting.
3. Major reactions: those that interfere with the examination and require treatment, e.g. severe bronchospasm, angioneurotic oedema.

The subcutaneous injection of contrast medium is painful and conventional contrast media have provoked sloughing of skin. This latter complication has not been reported with LOCM.

Renal size

Renal size, in particular length along the longest axis, may be measured and related to age, height or weight. We have found the method of Eklöf and Ringertz (1976a) to be the most useful. It relates renal length to the distance between the top of the body of the first lumbar vertebra and the bottom of the third lumbar vertebral body (Figures 9.1 and 9.2).

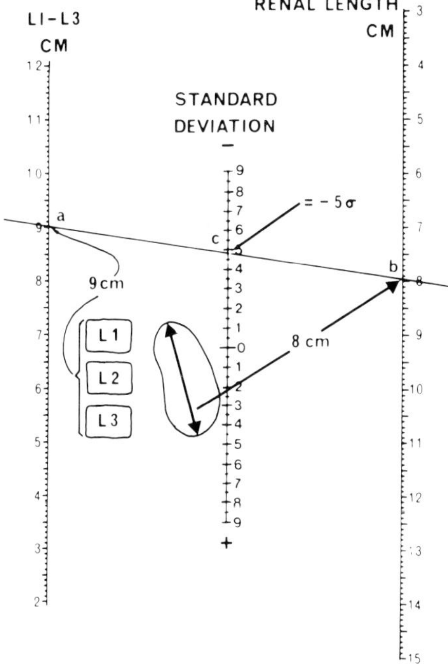

Figure 9.2 The method in practice. The length of the selected kidney is − 5 SD (From Eklöf and Ringertz, 1976a, by kind permission of the authors and publishers)

A quicker method of relating kidney size to vertebral body height is described by Currarino (1985). In the newborn kidney length is equivalent to the height of the five lumbar vertebral bodies and their intervening disc spaces. During the first 18 months of life the relationship is four and a half vertebral bodies and later in childhood the first four lumbar vertebral bodies and disc spaces, plus or minus 1 cm.

Following unilateral nephrectomy, the contralateral kidney undergoes prompt compensatory hypertrophy over the next 2 years. Compensatory hypertrophy of the normal kidney in children with unilateral renal agenesis or multicystic kidney only develops after birth (Eklöf and Ringertz, 1976b).

The normal urogram

The normal kidney contains 8–18 renal pyramids which terminate as papillae which indent the calyces. More than one pyramid may drain to a single papilla and although there is usually only one papilla to each calyx it is not uncommon to see a calyx with more than one papilla (a compound calyx). These compound calyces are most common in the poles and more commonly allow intrarenal reflux to occur, thus explaining why scarring due to reflux nephropathy is more common in both poles. Between the pyramids are extensions of renal cortex called the columns or septa of Bertin. A large column of Bertin will displace adjacent calyces and simulate a renal neoplasm (renal pseudotumour). Ultrasonography shows this tissue to be similar to normal renal cortex and a Tc-DMSA scan shows increased accumulation at that site (Parker et al., 1976).

If a line is drawn to connect the tips of the renal papillae (the interpapillary line of Hodson) then this line parallels the outer margin of the kidney (see Figure 9.6, p. 83) but with the upper and lower poles having a little more parenchyma than the mid-part. Even in the presence of normal variations of renal contour such as the dromedary hump or splenic or hepatic impressions on the renal contour, the arc of the interpapillary line maintains its parallel relationship with the renal contour. The presence of renal scarring may be recognized by approximation of the outer border of the kidney and the interpapillary line. On each side the distance of the medial upper-pole calyx from the midline is the same. Unilateral decrease is a further sign which suggests parenchymal loss (Friedland, Filly and Brown, 1974) while unilateral increase suggests the presence of a displacing mass, the most common pathological cause of the latter being a dilated ureter from a non-functioning, hydronephrotic, obstructed upper moiety of a duplex kidney. Fetal lobulation may persist after birth and presents as depressions of the renal outline which are sited between calyces and are not associated with deformity of adjacent calyces.

The kidneys lie in the retroperitoneum with their upper poles more medial and posterior than the lower poles. Because the lower-pole calyces are less dependent than the upper-pole calyces they may be less well opacified by contrast medium, which has a higher specific gravity than urine. Non-opacification of lower-pole calyces should not be assumed to be due to disease without a prone film which should remedy this unequal opacification. The normal renal pelvis may be large or small and lie within the renal sinus (intrarenal pelvis) or outside it (extrarenal pelvis). The pelvis divides into two or

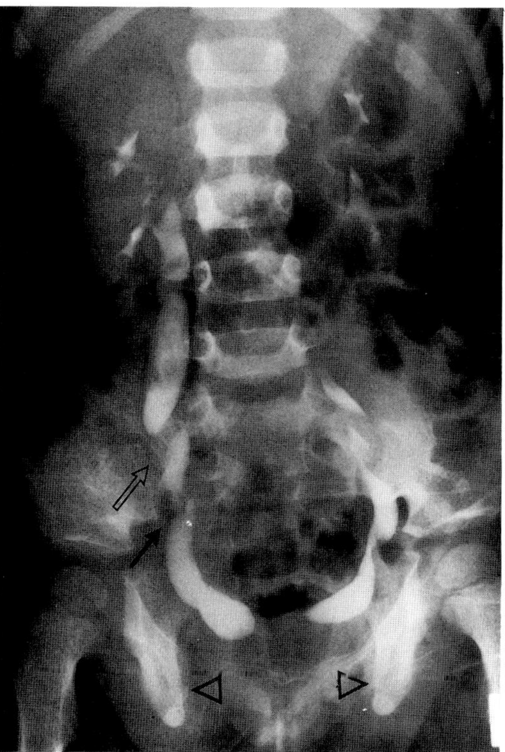

Figure 9.3 Vascular impressions are present at the right pelvi-ureteric junction and both ureters. Common iliac artery (*top arrow*) and common iliac vein (*bottom arrow*). Note also the widening of the symphysis pubis (*double arrows*) in this child with ectopia vesicae. Both ureters are dilated and obstructed at the uretero-vesical junctions

three major calyces which divide further into 8–12 minor calyces. Calyces are cup-like and the forniceal angles remain sharp unless there is increased pressure within the calyces or loss of papillary volume (see Figure 9.8, p. 86). The infundibulum of a calyx or the pelvi-ureteric junction may be indented by a renal artery (Kreel and Pyle, 1962) and rarely a true obstruction may develop. Oblique indentations on the ureters at the pelvic brim may also be observed due to underlying iliac vessels (Figure 9.3). Ureteric peristalsis quickly empties the normal ureter and it is unusual to see a ureter in its entirety on a single, full-length film during EU. Some dilatation of the upper tracts may occur with a distended bladder (Berdon and Baker, 1974; Gill and Curtis, 1977).

It is not uncommon to see a jet of opacified urine emerging from a ureteric orifice and hitting the opposite wall of the bladder (Figure 9.4). Vesico-ureteric reflux (VUR) is unlikely in children showing

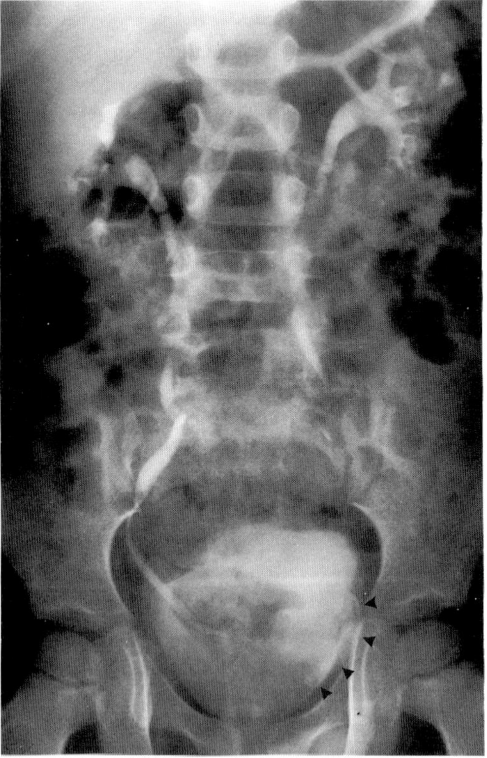

Figure 9.4 Ureteric jet issuing from the right ureteric opening and producing a cloud of contrast medium (*arrows*) when it strikes against the opposite wall of the bladder

this ureteric jet phenomenon (Kuhns *et al.*, 1977; Eklöf and Johanson, 1980).

The abnormal urogram

It is not the purpose of this book to discuss at length all the possible examples of urinary tract pathology that may be encountered. This section is intended to be a synopsis of the most commonly occurring conditions.

Non-visualization of one kidney

1. Nephrectomy: appropriate history and scar; $+/-$ partial resection of the 12th rib.
2. Agenesis: compensatory hypertrophy of contralateral kidney.
3. Multicystic/dysplastic kidney: may be a palpable renal mass.
4. Ectopic kidney: most commonly pelvic but may be thoracic.
5. Chronic obstruction: delayed films (up to 24 hours) may show some excretion.
6. Wilm's tumour.
7. Infection: pyelonephritis, pyonephrosis, tuberculosis or xantho-granulomatous pyelonephritis.

   Ultrasonography should be the next investigation and will either be diagnostic, e.g. revealing the presence of a multicystic kidney, or will determine the nature of subsequent investigations.

1. Dilatation of the pelvicalyceal system and/or ureter indicates obstruction or VUR although the latter only rarely results in complete non-function.
2. A solid mass may be further evaluated by computed tomography (CT).
3. An ultrasonically normal kidney indicates an inflammatory or vascular pathology.
4. Tc-DMSA scan may be necessary to differentiate renal agenesis from renal ectopia as the latter is often difficult to locate with US.

Nephrographic patterns (Newhouse and Pfister, 1979)

Immediate faint persistent nephrogram
1. Acute glomerulonephritis.
2. Renal vein thrombosis.
3. Severe chronic ischaemia.

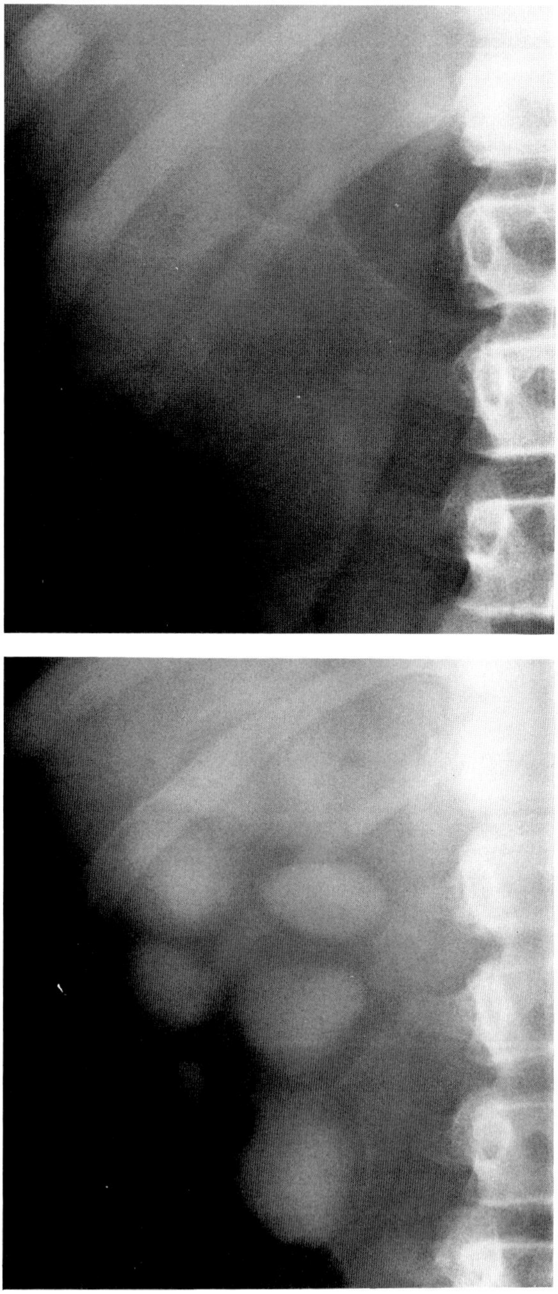

(a)

(b)

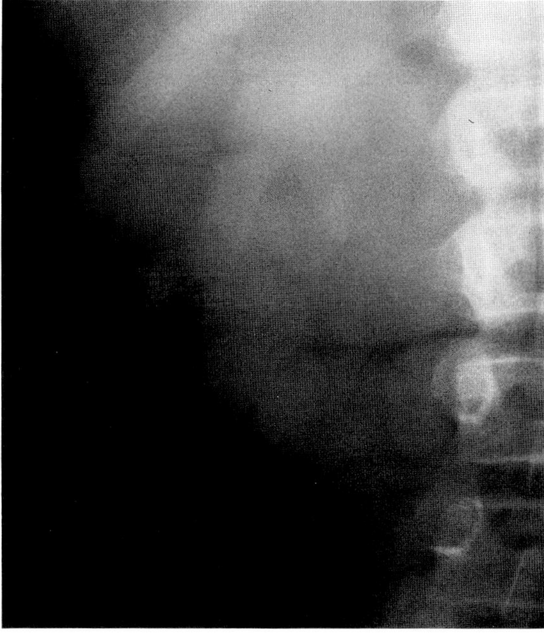

(c)

Figure 9.5 Severe hydronephrosis. (a) The earliest film from the urogram series shows contrast medium within the tubules of a thinned renal parenchyma resulting in the 'shell' or 'rim' nephrogram. At this early stage contrast medium has not reached the dilated calyces which still contain urine only. They, therefore, appear as filling defects within the opacified parenchyma – 'the negative pyelogram'. (b) When the dense contrast medium reaches the dilated calyces it will layer and the appearance will be that of puddles of contrast medium with the urine above. (c) As more contrast medium enters the calyces urine is displaced and further mixing occurs. Ultimately the entire pelvicalyceal system becomes opacified

Immediate distinct persistent nephrogram
1. Acute renal failure: especially acute tubular necrosis.
2. Acute-on-chronic renal failure.
3. Acute hypotension.

Increasingly dense nephrogram
1. Acute obstruction: including urate nephropathy.
2. Acute hypotension.
3. Acute tubular necrosis: in 30% of cases.
4. Acute pyelonephritis.
5. Renal vein thrombosis.
6. Acute glomerulonephritis.

Rim nephrogram
1. Severe hydronephrosis: a shell of squashed parenchyma is followed, on delayed films, by puddles of contrast medium in dilated calyces and, later still, by homogeneous opacification of calyces and pelvis (Figure 9.5).

Striated nephrogram
1. Infantile polycystic disease.
2. Acute ureteric obstruction.
3. Acute pyelonephritis.
4. Medullary sponge kidney.

Unilateral scarred kidney

See Figure 9.6 and Davidson (1977i).

Unilateral small smooth kidney

Note: the left kidney may normally be a little smaller than the right. In conditions with chronic unilateral renal disease there will be compensatory hypertrophy of the contralateral kidney.

With a dilated collecting system
Post-obstructive atrophy – with generalized cortical thinning and impaired excretion of contrast medium.

With a small-volume collecting system
Renal ischaemia – small-volume collecting system suggests diminished urine volume and in association with cortical thinning and delayed but dense opacification of calyces indicates ischaemia.

With five or less calyces
Hypoplasia – normal pelvicalyceal system and normal function.

See also Davidson (1977ii).

Unilateral large smooth kidney

1. Compensatory hypertrophy.
2. Duplex kidney.
3. Chronic hydronephrosis, pyonephrosis: poor or no function.
4. Multicystic kidney: no function. May be contralateral pelvi-ureteric junction obstruction. Ultrasonography reveals multiple cysts which do not communicate.

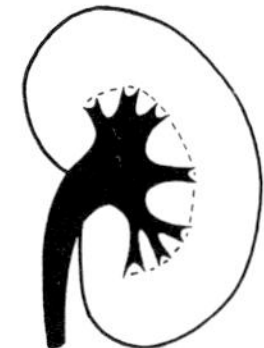

NORMAL
Cortex parallel to
interpapillary line

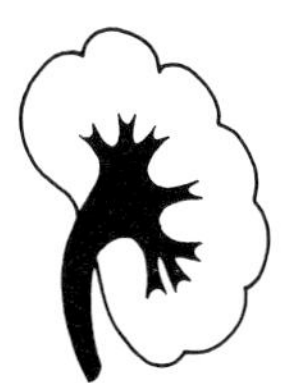

FETAL LOBULATION
Normal size. Cortical
depressions between
papillae

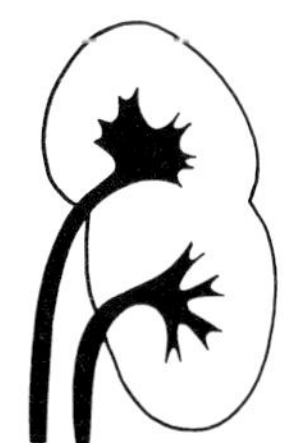

DUPLEX KIDNEY
Renal size usually
larger than normal

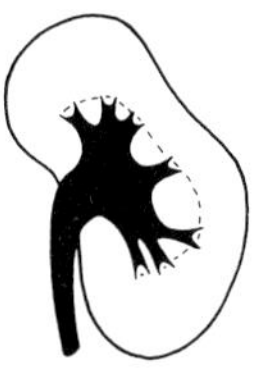

SPLEEN IMPRESSION
Right kidney may
show hepatic
impression

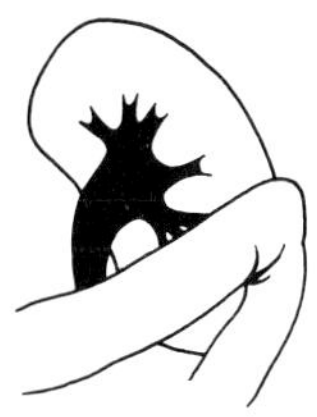

OVERLYING BOWEL
Spurious loss of
cortex

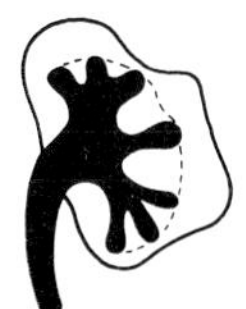

REFLUX
NEPHROPATHY
Focal scars over
dilated calyces. Most
prominent at upper
and lower poles. May
be bilateral

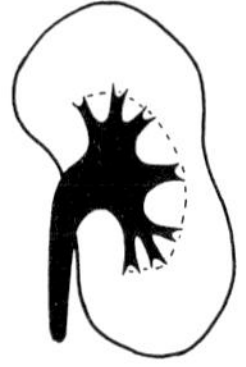

LOBAR INFARCTION
Broad depression
over a normal calyx

Figure 9.6 Scarred kidney. Diagrammatic representation of EU appearances in some conditions associated with cortical depressions. The changes could be unilateral or bilateral.

5. Wilms' tumour: usually a few residual calyces do opacify but are displaced and distorted.
6. Crossed ectopia: one ureter crosses the midline. No contralateral kidney.

7. Acute pyelonephritis: impaired excretion, attenuated calyces $+/-$ increasingly dense or striated nephrogram. Abnormality may be focal.
8. Renal vein thrombosis: sudden onset – a large non-functioning kidney which over a period of several weeks or months may atrophy. If thrombosis is gradual function is preserved but with attenuation of calyces and there may be ureteric notching due to venous collaterals.
9. Acute arterial infarction.

See also Davidson (1977iii).

Bilateral large smooth kidneys

1. Bilateral hydronephrosis.
2. Polycystic disease.
3. Renal vein thrombosis.
4. Visceromegaly: gigantism, Beckwith–Wiedemann syndrome.
5. Proliferative/necrotizing disorders.
6. Leukaemic/lymphomatous infiltration.
7. Acute interstitial nephritis.
8. Acute tubular necrosis.

Radiological differentiation between these conditions is seldom possible. Clinical and biochemical features are more helpful.

See also Davidson (1977iv).

Renal space-occupying lesions

See Figure 9.7.

Hydronephrosis

Clubbing of the calyces is due to increased intraluminal pressure or deformity from scarring. The sequence of changes is illustrated in Figure 9.8.

Obstruction

AT THE INFUNDIBULUM OF A CALYX
1. An intrarenal artery: commonly an upper pole calyx (Fraley syndrome).
2. Calculus, tuberculosis, tumour.

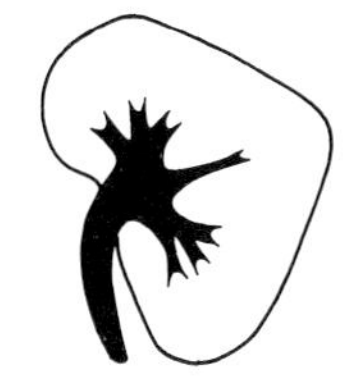

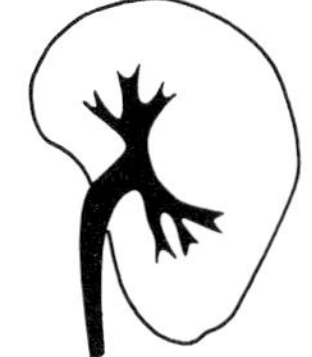

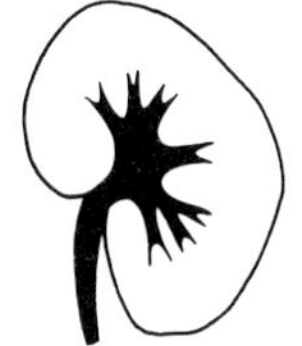

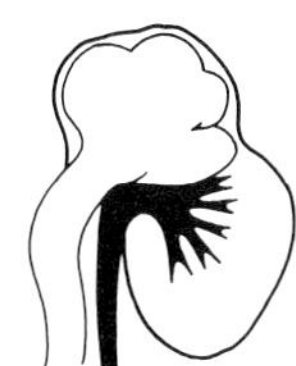

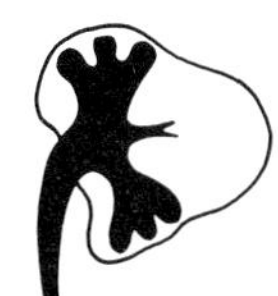

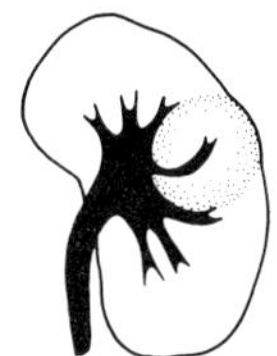

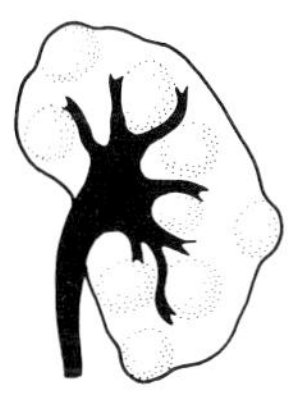

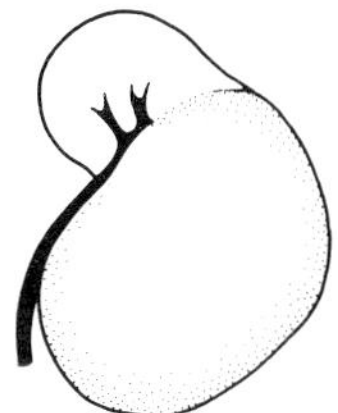

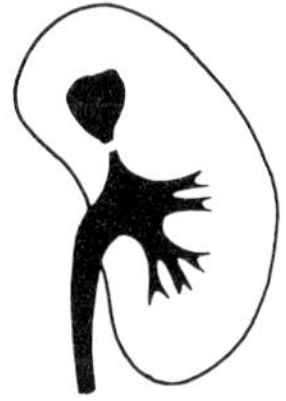

Figure 9.7 Space-occupying lesion. Diagrammatic representation of EU appearances in some conditions associated with a renal mass(es)

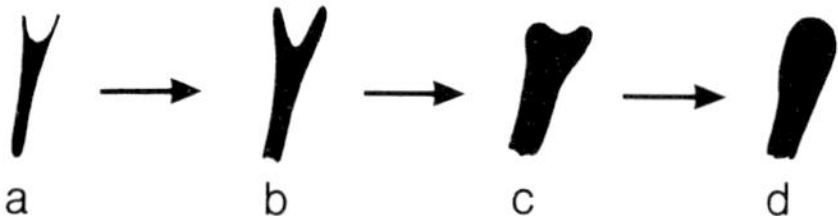

Figure 9.8 Stages in the development of a hydrocalyx. (a) The normal calyx with a prominent papilla and sharp fornices. (b) Blunting of the forniceal angles.
(c) Rounding of the fornices and a poor impression by the papilla. (d) A clubbed calyx with complete loss of fornices and papilla

AT THE PELVI-URETERIC JUNCTION

1. Idiopathic.
2. Renal artery.

URETERIC

1. Congenital megaureter: most commonly at the uretero-vesical junction. Reflux may also occur.
2. Ureterocoele: either from a single system kidney or on the upper moiety ureter of a duplex kidney. The latter has an ectopic orifice, either in the bladder or outside it, e.g. vagina.
3. Ectopic ureter.
4. Calculus.
5. Extrinsic compression: faecal loading of rectosigmoid, tumour or a retrocaval ureter.

WITHIN THE BLADDER

1. Neurogenic bladder.
2. Tumour: usually a rhabdomyosarcoma.
3. Ureterocoele: a very large ureterocoele may obstruct the contra-lateral ureter.

DISTAL TO THE BLADDER

1. Posterior urethral valves: males.
2. Ectopic ureterocoele.
3. Urethral stricture: most frequently post-traumatic.
4. Diverticulum.
5. Prune belly syndrome: dysplastic posterior urethra.
6. Calculus or foreign body.
7. Meatal stenosis. ⎫
8. Phimosis. ⎬ Clinical diagnoses.
　　　　　　　　⎭

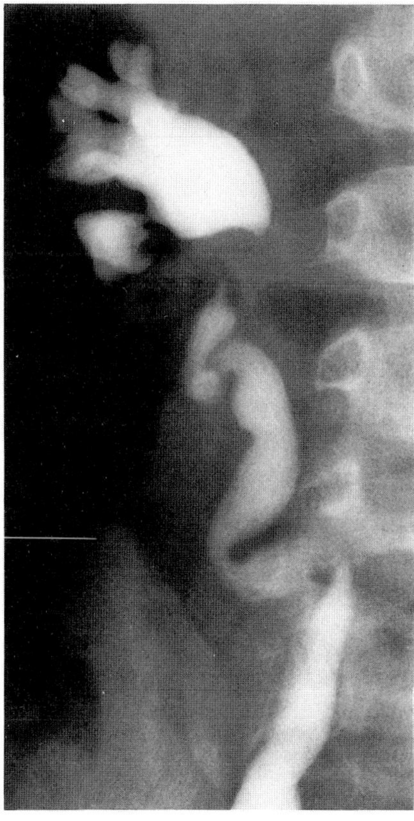

Figure 9.9 Ureteric striations

Reflux

1. Without scarring: renal cortex is preserved. Longitudinal striations in the ureter (Figure 9.9) suggest the presence of reflux even in the absence of dilatation.
2. With scarring: calyceal clubbing is now due to distortion from parenchymal fibrosis and is not reversible. There is loss of cortex overlying the dilated calyces but this may be difficult to detect at the upper and lower poles where cortex is normally thicker than elsewhere.

Atonia

1. Following the relief of an obstruction.
2. During an infection.
3. Prune belly syndrome.

Micturating cystourethrography

Fluoroscopically monitored micturating cystourethrography (MCUG) is the definitive method of studying the anatomy of the lower urinary tract.

Indications

1. To determine if vesico-ureteric reflux is occurring in a child with urinary tract infection.
2. To determine if vesico-ureteric reflux is occurring in a child who has been shown to have hydroureteronephrosis by US or EU.
3. Small kidneys or renal failure of undetermined cause.
4. Disturbance of micturition. In boys this may be due to structural abnormalities such as posterior urethral valves. Structural abnormalities in girls are rare but contrast cystography may be performed as part of a urodynamics investigation (see Chapter 12).
5. Haematuria with lower urinary tract symptoms.

Contraindications

1. Urinary tract infection. Conventional teaching says that several weeks should elapse after the urine has become sterile so that vesico-ureteric reflux secondary to infection has time to resolve. Reflux is not usually secondary to infection although the presence of gram-negative bacterial endotoxins which reduce urinary tract tone may make pre-existing reflux appear more severe. The argument in favour of early MCUG is that if reflux does only occur in the presence of infection then that would be useful information to know as it is the reflux of infected urine that results in renal scarring. Lebowitz (1985) argues that in practice MCUG may be performed when it is most convenient but the authors still prefer to wait several weeks after the commencement of chemotherapy. The risk from introduction of new infection is small provided catheterization is performed with aseptic technique and the child should remain on antibiotics from the time of diagnosis until investigations are complete.

Technique

If possible the child micturates prior to the examination so that contrast medium is not diluted by a large volume of urine in the bladder. Anxiety will be alleviated by carefully explaining the procedure to the parents and child and catheterization should be performed by someone skilled in such a procedure. Sedation is to be avoided. Using aseptic technique a lubricated catheter (a 5–8 F feeding tube is satisfactory) is advanced through the urethra into the bladder and fixed in position by adhesive tape. Residual urine is drained. When catheterization of the male urethra is difficult it is advisable to perform a retrograde urethrogram to exclude an obstruction. If the urethra is normal but the bladder still cannot be entered the bladder can either be filled by instilling contrast medium directly into the urethra and pinching the meatus or, in a baby, by performing a suprapubic puncture.

Any water-soluble contrast medium with a concentration of iodine of approximately $150\,mg\,ml^{-1}$ (Urografin 150, Hypaque 25%) is satisfactory. It is dripped into the bladder and filling is monitored by fluoroscopy. Any VUR is recorded on film. The catheter should not be removed until the radiologist is convinced the child will micturate or no more contrast medium will drip into the bladder. When micturition commences the catheter is quickly withdrawn. Young children can lie on the table to micturate but older children will find it easier to stand. In infants and children with a neuropathic bladder micturition may be initiated by suprapubic pressure. The following films are taken:

1. Full bladder in the frontal projection.
2. A 45° oblique view of the bladder and urethra during micturition. In boys the oblique projection is necessary to prevent radiographic foreshortening of the urethra. It will also reveal reflux into the lower end of the ureter on the side that is elevated so that prior knowledge of one side being abnormal will determine which oblique will be necessary.
3. Post-micturition film of the abdomen to include bladder and renal areas to demonstrate any reflux of contrast medium into the kidneys that might have occurred unnoticed and to record bladder residue.

Aftercare

Parents should be advised that dysuria, occasionally leading to retention of urine, may occur. The administration of a simple analgesic is usually all that is necessary. If the child is receiving antibiotics following a urinary tract infection these should be continued until the results of the investigation are reviewed.

Complications

The majority of complications are related to poor catheterization technique, i.e. introduction of infection and trauma to the urethra. A very traumatic catheterization may create a false passage or initiate a stricture but this is rare. Occasionally the vagina or an ectopic urethral orifice is catheterized but this can be recognized by fluoroscopic monitoring when contrast medium is first instilled.

Grading of vesico-ureteric reflux

Vesico-ureteric reflux (VUR) presents a spectrum of severity which may vary not only between examinations but also within a single examination. Differences in severity may be due to:

1. Maturation of the vesico-ureteric junction with age.
2. Differences in bladder filling.
3. The technique of MCUG (filling with a syringe may affect bladder filling and voiding) (Lebowitz *et al.*, 1985).

A number of grading systems based on the radiographic appearances at MCUG are in operation. An international system (Lebowitz *et al.*, 1985) has been proposed and is summarized below.

Grade I: Ureter only.
Grade II: Ureter, pelvis and calyces; no dilatation and normal fornices.
Grade III: Mild or moderate dilatation and/or tortuosity of the ureter and mild or moderate dilatation of the renal pelvis. No or slight blunting of the fornices.

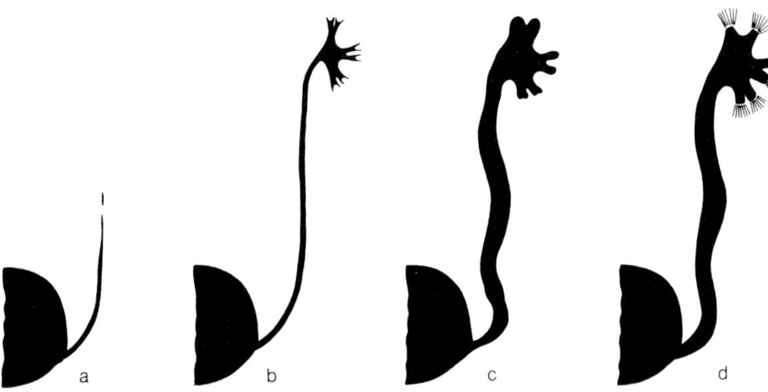

Figure 9.10 Grading of vesico-ureteric reflux. (a) Grade I: into the ureter only, without dilatation. (b) Grade II: into the ureter, pelvis and calyces, without dilatation. (c) Grade III: into the ureter, pelvis and calyces, with dilatation. (d) As with (c) but with intrarenal reflux

Grade IV: Moderate dilatation and/or tortuosity of the ureter and moderate dilatation of the renal pelvis and calyces. The sharp angle of the fornices is lost but papillary impressions in the majority of calyces are maintained.

Grade V: Gross dilatation of the ureter, calyces and pelvis. The papillary impressions are no longer visible.

We have used a simplified classification which is illustrated diagrammatically in Figure 9.10. The grade is determined by the most severe VUR during the procedure and this usually coincides with the peak of voiding when bladder pressure is at its highest.

Ascending urethrography

Retrograde injection of contrast medium into the male urethra is the method to be employed for evaluation of abnormalities of the anterior urethra. This technique does not produce adequate distension of the posterior urethra because of spasm of the external sphincter; MCUG should be employed for imaging the posterior urethra. Using aseptic technique a feeding catheter or balloon catheter is inserted into the distal anterior urethra. The meatus is occluded either by the firm application of adhesive tape or by carefully inflating the balloon, which is positioned in the fossa navicularis. The patient is turned into a 45° oblique position and films exposed while contrast medium is injected under fluoroscopic control.

Complications include the introduction of infection, urethral trauma and the intravasation of contrast medium if excessive pressure is used to overcome a stricture.

Retrograde pyelo-ureterography

With modern imaging techniques such as US and isotope renography and high quality EU the indications for retrograde urography have decreased. The most frequent indication today is to demonstrate, prior to surgery, the exact site of obstruction in a known case of obstructive hydronephrosis, most commonly pelvi-ureteric junction obstruction when the ureter has not been demonstrated by US or EU. Under general anaesthesia the urologist introduces a catheter via a cystoscope into the ureter or renal pelvis and films are exposed during the injection of contrast medium. The entire procedure usually takes place in one site, i.e. the operating theatre or the X-ray department. Occasionally the catheter may be introduced in the operating theatre, taped in position and later, with the patient awake, contrast medium is injected by the radiologist and films exposed in the X-ray department.

Antegrade percutaneous studies

Antegrade pyelography is indicated in the following circumstances:

1. When less invasive tests such as diuretic renography have failed to differentiate obstructive from non-obstructive upper tract dilatation and if obstructed, at what level and from what cause. In this situation imaging is often combined with perfusion pressure flow measurements – the Whitaker test (Whitaker, 1973; Pfister, 1982).
2. When less invasive tests have failed to differentiate multicystic kidney from hydronephrosis due to pelvi-ureteric junction obstruction. In the former there are discrete cysts whereas in the latter the 'cysts' are dilated calyces and pelvis which communicate with each other.
3. Prior to percutaneous nephrostomy or other interventional procedures (Lang, 1986).

Defects in coagulation are an absolute contraindication to percutaneous renal puncture. General anaesthesia or sedation will be required and the age of the child together with his or her ability to cooperate will determine which is used. The collecting system is localized by US, CT or following intravenous injection of contrast medium, the choice being determined by personal preference and renal function. Only US and CT are applicable when renal function is poor and US is the method of choice. Using aseptic technique the kidney is punctured using a long thin needle with a stylette. When urine is obtained the needle is correctly sited. Aspirated urine is sent for microscopy and culture. Contrast medium is injected under fluoroscopic control and films exposed of the relevant anatomy and abnormality.

When there are continuing concerns about the presence of an obstruction the needle can be connected to equipment that will infuse contrast medium and measure renal pelvic pressure. A catheter in the bladder is used to determine bladder pressure, VUR having already been excluded by a previous MCUG. *Absolute* renal pressure and *relative* pressure (bladder pressure subtracted from renal pressure) can be measured. In the normal urinary tract infusion of a dilute contrast medium at a rate of $10\,\text{ml}\,\text{min}^{-1}$ produces a relative pressure in the renal pelvis less than $15\,\text{cm}\ H_2O$ above that in the bladder. Pressures greater than $22\,\text{cm}\ H_2O$ indicate obstruction while $15\text{–}22\,\text{cm}\ H_2O$ are in the equivocal range (Whitaker, 1979).

Temporary relief of upper tract obstruction may be obtained by percutaneous nephrostomy. The collecting system is identified by EU (if renal function is adequate), US or antegrade pyelography. The puncture point is chosen on the posterior axillary line below the 12th rib. A needle wide enough to take a guide wire is introduced through the skin, subcutaneous tissues and renal parenchyma into the renal pelvis. When correctly sited in the renal pelvis the stylette is withdrawn and a guide wire threaded through the needle into the pelvis. The needle is withdrawn and a series of dilators passed over the wire to dilate the tract. Finally a pigtail catheter is introduced over the wire, the wire is removed and the catheter is secured to the skin (Irving, Arthur and Thomas, 1987).

Loopogram

It may be necessary to study the ileal loop of those patients who have had an ileal loop diversion. The ureters are usually implanted without an antireflux procedure so reflux is to be expected. In these patients a deterioration of upper tract dilatation and/or renal function may be due to stomal or ureteric obstruction. A balloon catheter is introduced into the loop and urine drained to determine the residual urine volume. Contrast medium is injected under fluoroscopic control and spot films taken. Known dilatation of the upper tracts in the absence of ileo-ureteric reflux suggests obstruction at the anastomosis. The stoma is best viewed in a tangential projection following removal of the catheter and obstruction is suggested by a large loop which drains poorly.

Arteriography

Indications

1. Hypertension.
2. Prior to conservative surgical treatment of Wilms' tumour, particularly bilateral tumours.
3. For the detailed visualization of small vessel renal disease.
4. Prior to interventional procedures on the kidney, e.g. percutaneous renal artery angioplasty.

Technique

Arteriography is not an investigation to be undertaken lightly and should only be performed by an operator skilled in the technique as it applies to children. Depending on the age of the child and the degree of cooperation to be expected the investigation will be performed under general anaesthesia or sedation and strict asepsis is observed. The technique of catheter placement in a vessel is known as the Seldinger technique, after the Swedish radiologist who developed it (Seldinger, 1953), and is outlined in diagrammatic form in Figure 9.11. The catheter is most frequently introduced by the transfemoral route and advanced under fluoroscopic control to lie either in the abdominal aorta or in a renal artery. For the aortogram a straight catheter with multiple side-holes is most suitable while for selective catheterization of a renal artery a catheter with a preformed curve at its tip and an end-hole is used.

We have not found that a venous injection of contrast medium and manipulation of the images by digital subtraction techniques give adequate detail.

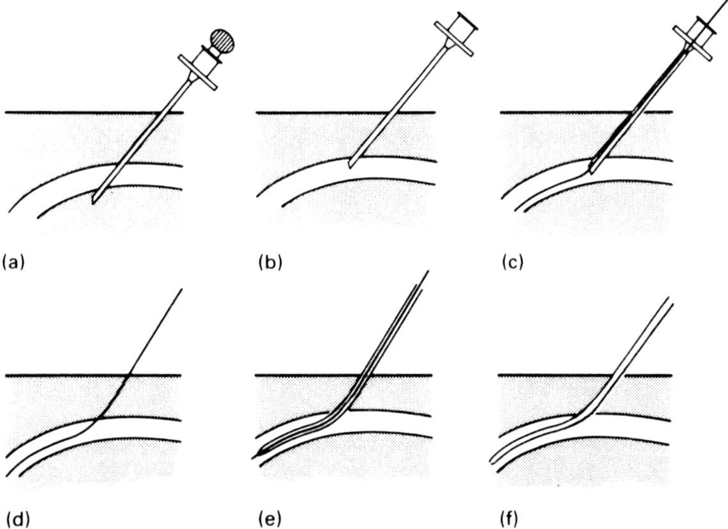

Figure 9.11 Seldinger technique for introducing an angiographic catheter into an artery or vein. (a) Both walls of the vessel are punctured. (b) The stilette is removed; the needle is withdrawn and when the bevel enters the lumen of the vessel blood flows from the hub. (c) The guide wire is passed through the needle. (d) The needle is withdrawn leaving the guide wire *in situ*. (e) The catheter is threaded over the wire. (f) The guide wire is withdrawn (From Chapman and Nakielny, 1986, by permission of the publishers)

Venography and renal vein sampling

Venography and renal vein sampling for plasma renin activity (PRA) are undertaken prior to possible surgical correction of renin-dependent hypertension and are usually performed at the same time as arteriography. Using the Seldinger technique a preshaped catheter is introduced into the femoral vein and passed to the inferior vena cava, both renal veins and the segmental renal veins. Plasma renin activity is assayed in blood sampled from all these sites and when the ratio between the two kidneys exceeds 1.5:1 renin-dependent hypertension is confirmed. Excessively high levels from a particular segmental vein will indicate that partial rather than total nephrectomy may be possible.

Computed tomography

Computed tomography (CT) detects X-ray attenuation differences of tissues and by computer analysis of these differences is able to display cross-sectional images of the body. Routine scanning produces images in the axial plane but it is possible to reconstruct the data into other image planes. Because motion degrades image quality the patient must be still during scanning and young children will need sedation or even general anaesthesia. Contrast resolution is improved by intravenous contrast medium enhancement, the type and dosage being similar to those employed for EU. Bowel loops may mimic solid masses or abscesses and for this reason oral or rectal contrast enhancement is frequently employed. Dilute intravenous contrast medium or dilute barium sulphate is satisfactory for this purpose.

Computed tomography of the abdomen and pelvis is most often indicated for the further investigation of mass lesions, particularly neoplasms. Initial investigation is likely to be with US and/or EU but CT excells at demonstrating the extent of disease, is more sensitive to the presence of calcification and by revealing specific tissue components such as fat may suggest diagnoses such as teratoma or angiomyolipoma (a rare renal tumour occurring almost exclusively in patients with tuberous sclerosis). Blunt abdominal trauma provides a further indication, especially when injury to more than one organ is suspected. Computed tomography is also more sensitive for the detection of nephrocalcinosis and renal calculi and in the latter situation the improved anatomical localization of a calyceal calculus may be of benefit to the surgeon (Berger *et al.*, 1980).

References and further reading

Excretion urography

Currarino, G. (1985) The genitourinary tract. In *Caffey's Paediatric X-Ray Diagnosis*, 8th edn, Vol. 2 (ed. F. N. Silverman), Year Book Medical Publishers, Chicago, p. 1611

Dawson, P. (1985) Contrast agent nephrotoxicity. An appraisal. *British Journal of Radiology*, **58**, 121–124

Eklöf, O. and Ringertz, H. (1976a) Kidney size in children: a method of assessment. *Acta Radiologica [Diagnosis] (Stockholm)*, **17**, 617–625

Eklöf, O. and Ringertz, H. (1976b) Kidney size and growth in unilateral renal agenesis and in the remaining kidney following nephrectomy for Wilms' tumour. *Acta Radiologica [Diagnosis] (Stockholm)*, **17**, 601–608

Gerber, W. L. and Brown, R. C. (1985) The value of post-void radiographs in excretion urography. *Clinical Radiology*, **36**, 525–527

Grainger, R. G. (1984) The clinical and financial implications of the low-osmolar contrast media. *Clinical Radiology*, **35**, 251–252

Hope, J. W. and Campoy, F. (1955). The use of carbonated beverages in paediatric excretory urography. *Radiology*, **64**, 66–71

Manhire, A. R., Dawson, P. and Dennet, R. (1984) Contrast agent induced emesis. *Clinical Radiology*, **35**, 369–370

Rao, V. M., Rao, A. K., Steiner, R. M., Burka, E. R., Grainger, R. G. and Ballas, S. K. (1982) The effect of ionic and nonionic contrast media on the sickling phenomenon. *Radiology*, **144**, 291–293

Spataro, R. F. (1984) Newer contrast agents for urography. *Radiologic Clinics of North America*, **22**, 365–380

The normal urogram

Berdon, W. E. and Baker, D. H. (1974) The significance of a distended bladder in the interpretation of intravenous pyelograms obtained on patients with 'hydronephrosis'. *American Journal of Roentgenology*, **120**, 402–409

Eklöf, O. A. and Johanson, L. (1980) Occurrence of reflux in children with ureteral jets. *Paediatric Radiology*, **10**, 95–99

Friedland, G. W., Filly, R. and Brown, B. W. (1974) Distance of upper pole calyx to spine and lower pole calyx to ureter as indicators of parenchymal loss in children. *Paediatric Radiology*, **2**, 29–37

Gill, W. B. and Curtis, G. A. (1977) The influence of bladder fullness on upper urinary tract dimensions and renal excretory function. *Journal of Urology*, **117**, 573–576

Kreel, L. and Pyle, R. (1962) Arterial impression on the renal pelvis. *British Journal of Radiology*, **35**, 609–613

Kuhns, L. R., Hernandez, R., Koff, S. *et al.* (1977) Absence of vesicoureteral reflux in children with ureteral jets. *Radiology*, **124**, 185–187

Parker, J. A., Lebowitz, R. L., Mascatello, V. and Treves, S. (1976) Magnification renal scintigraphy in the differential diagnosis of septa of Bertin. *Paediatric Radiology*, **4**, 157–160

The abnormal urogram

Davidson, A. J. (1977) *Radiologic Diagnosis of Renal Parenchymal Disease*, W. B. Saunders, Philadelphia, (i) chap. 4; (ii) chap. 5; (iii) chap. 8; (iv) chap. 7.

Newhouse, J. H. and Pfister, R. C. (1979) The nephrogram. *Radiologic Clinics of North America*, **17**, 213–226

Micturating cystourethrography

Lebowitz, R. L. (1985) Paediatric uradiology. *Pediatric Clinics of North America*, **32**, 1353–1362

Grading of vesico-ureteric reflux

Lebowitz, R. L., Olbing, H., Parkkulainen, K. V. *et al.* (1985) International system of grading of vesico-ureteric reflux. *Paediatric Radiology*, **15**, 105–109

Antegrade percutaneous studies

Irving, H. C., Arthur, R. J. and Thomas, D. F. M. (1987) Percutaneous nephrostomy in paediatrics. *Clinical Radiology*, **38**, 245–248

Lang, E. K. (ed.) (1986) Interventional uroradiology. *Radiologic Clinics of North America*, **24**, no. 4

Pfister, R. C. (1982) Pressure flow studies II. In *Idiopathic Hydronephrosis* (eds P. H. O'Reilly and J. A. Gosling), Springer, Berlin, pp. 68–78

Whitaker, R. H. (1973) Methods of assessing obstruction in dilated ureters. *British Journal of Urology*, **45**, 15–22

Whitaker, R. H. (1979) An evaluation of 170 diagnostic pressure flow studies in the upper urinary tract. *Journal of Urology*, **121**, 602–604

Loopogram

Koehler, P. R. and Bowles, W. T. (1973) Radiologic evaluation of the upper urinary tract following ileal loop urinary diversion. *Radiology*, **86**, 227–234

Arteriography

Chapman, S. and Nakielny, R. A. (1986) *Guide to Radiological Procedures*, 2nd edn, Baillière Tindall, London, chap. 8

Kirks, D. R., Fitz, C. R. and Harwood-Nash, D. C. (1976) Paediatric abdominal angiography: practical guide to catheter selection, flow rates and contrast dosage. *Paediatric Radiology*, **5**, 19–23

Seldinger, S. (1953) Catheter replacement of needle in percutaneous arteriography: new technique. *Acta Radiologica*, **39**, 368–376

Computed tomography

Berger, P. E., Munschauer, F. W. and Kuhn, J. P. (1980) Computed tomography and ultrasound of renal and perirenal diseases in infants and children. *Paediatric Radiology*, **9**, 91–99

Kirks, D. R. (1983a) Computed tomography of paediatric urinary tract disease. *Urologic Radiology*, **5**, 199–208

Kirks, D. R. (1983b) Practical techniques for paediatric computed tomography. *Pediatric Radiology*, **13**, 148–155

Kuhn, J. P. and Berger, P. E. (1981a) Computed tomography of the kidney in infancy and childhood. *Radiologic Clinics of North America*, **19**, 445–461

Kuhn, J. P. and Berger, P. E. (1981b) Computed tomography in the evaluation of blunt trauma in children. *Radiologic Clinics of North America*, **19**, 399–408

Siegel, M. J., Glasier, C. M. and Sagel, S. S. (1981) CT of pelvic disorders in children. *American Journal of Roentgenology*, **137**, 1139–1143

Chapter 10

Imaging: ultrasonography

Ultrasonography

Excretion urography (EU) has, over the years, been regarded as the most important tool for the investigation of the urinary tract and in complex cases it is often the one test that gives the best overall picture. With the advent of modern, high resolution, real-time ultrasound equipment EU has, for many problems, been progressively relegated to a secondary role; but whereas EU gives not only anatomical information but also a crude indication of function, ultrasonography (US) yields only anatomical information. Because US does not depend on excretion it can demonstrate anatomy even in the kidney without function. When US is used to delineate structure, information about renal function is usually obtained from radionuclide studies (see Chapter 11).

Indications (Lebowitz, 1985)

1. Urinary tract infection – to document scarring (Figure 10.1) and to exclude an underlying structural abnormality (Mason, 1984; Kangarloo *et al.*, 1985; Leonidas *et al.*, 1985; Lindsell and Moncrief, 1986).
2. An abdominal or pelvic mass. Ultrasonography will demonstrate the relationship of the mass to other organs, its possible site of origin and its characteristics, i.e. solid or cystic and presence of calcification.
3. Renal failure. Because US is not dependent on function it is ideal for differentiating medical from surgical causes of renal failure.
4. Abnormal antenatal ultrasound. To confirm or refute an antenatal diagnosis of hydronephrosis or cystic renal disease. The role of US should be to help in the efficient planning of the postnatal management before infection occurs and plasma creatinine rises rather than to provoke antenatal fetal intervention (Lebowitz and Teele, 1983). It must be remembered that

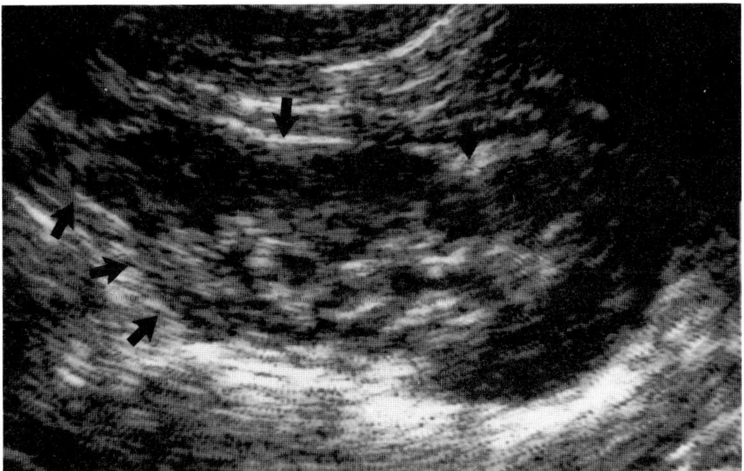

Figure 10.1 Longitudinal scan of a kidney showing renal scarring (*arrows*), most marked at the upper pole. (By convention, longitudinal scans are displayed with the head end of the patient on the left)

because urine output falls rapidly at birth when compared with urine output *in utero*, US on day 1 may show considerably less pelvicalyceal dilatation than was observed on the antenatal scans. Further follow-up US scans are mandatory.

5. To determine the site of obstruction when excretion urography has demonstrated obstructive uropathy but failed to localize the exact level (Chopra and Teele, 1980).

6. To evaluate a kidney that has not been visualized by EU or radionuclide studies.

7. Conditions which are associated with a high likelihood of renal anomalies. These include imperforate anus, genital anomalies, congenital vertebral anomalies and Fanconi's anaemia. The most frequently found abnormalities are single kidney and ectopic kidney.

8. Conditions which predispose to renal tumours (Miller, Fraumenti and Manning, 1964). Periodic screening is recommended in children with Beckwith–Wiedemann syndrome, hemihypertrophy and aniridia.

9. Screening of family members for genetically linked renal diseases, e.g. adult-type polycystic disease.

10. Periodic follow-up of kidneys which are at risk of deterioration, i.e. those children with a myelomeningocoele or a urinary diversion. Patients on chronic dialysis have a high incidence of

acquired cystic disease and may develop adenomas or adenocarcinomas.
11. To assess the patency of the inferior vena cava in patients with Wilm's tumour who may have tumour thrombus.
12. To assess residual bladder volume.
13. To facilitate the accurate placement of needles for renal biopsy, antegrade pyelography, percutaneous nephrostomy, cyst aspiration and the drainage of fluid collections in the perirenal space.

Technique

Real-time equipment rather than the now antiquated static B-mode scanners are indicated for paediatric use although an articulated arm, static B scanner may be necessary to measure the long axis of a kidney which is too large to be measured by a real-time sector scanner. Sedation is only rarely required. A short- or variable-focus 5-MHz transducer is recommended. In small babies a 7.5-MHz transducer gives improved resolution while in the larger teenager it may be necessary to use a 3.5-MHz or 2.5-MHz transducer to obtain the necessary penetration. A major limitation of US is the inability of the sound beam to penetrate air or bone. Bowel gas may limit access to the kidneys from the front of the abdomen while the lower ribs frequently obscure the upper poles of the kidneys when they are examined from the back. It is often difficult to obtain ideal renal images in patients with severe scoliosis.

If possible the patient should be examined with a full bladder so that the bladder can be used as an acoustic window to look at the lower ends of the ureters. Patients with an indwelling catheter should have the catheter clamped 1 hour before the examination. In babies it is advisable to begin by looking at the bladder first because contact with the transducer frequently initiates micturition and this may be the only opportunity to obtain images of it. If micturition occurs before adequate images are obtained or if the bladder is only partly full then it can be rescanned after the kidneys. The bladder is scanned in longitudinal and transverse planes and this is followed by longitudinal and transverse scans of the kidneys. If possible the kidneys are examined on full inspiration or with the child being asked to 'push the tummy out', this making the kidneys more accessible to the US beam. By scanning from the front satisfactory images of at least the upper two-thirds of the right kidney are possible and adjacent liver can be used as a reference for renal cortical echogenicity. The lower third of the right kidney and all of the left kidney are usually inaccessible from the front. Satisfactory images of the left kidney are possible from the back. When scanning with the patient prone the proximity of the lower ribs to the pelvic brim may be decreased by lying the child over a pillow. The authors take further images of the right kidney in the prone position. Scanning in the lateral decubitus position with the child on his or her side will produce coronal sections of each kidney comparable to those familiar on conventional radiographs.

The upper urinary tract

Normal anatomy

A number of anatomical features may be identified. In longitudinal sections (Figure 10.2) the kidney is ovoid in shape; in transverse sections (Figure 10.3) it resembles a doughnut above and below the hilum and a horseshoe at the hilum. The renal cortex is less echogenic than adjacent liver or spleen (the spleen being slightly less echogenic than liver). Centrally there are bright echoes from the calyceal walls and in the renal hilum bright echoes arise from the walls of the renal pelvis, renal artery and vein and parapelvic fat. The high echogenicity of the hilar region can occasionally obscure small calculi at this site. The calyces and infundibula are potential spaces and are frequently visualized as echolucent structures. The degree of calyceal wall separation is dependent on urine output and is more marked in the presence of a diuresis; minor separation is without significance. Renal pyramids are well-defined triangular structures which are more echolucent than adjacent cortex. The base of the triangle is cortical and the apex is in contact with the central bright calyceal echoes. Cortex extends between the pyramids as the septa of Bertin. The echogenic arcuate arteries define the corticomedullary junction. It is usually possible to demonstrate the renal arteries and veins, aorta and inferior vena cava.

The renal pelvis is identified at the hilum as an oval echolucent region with its long axis in a similar orientation to the long axis of the kidney. Like the calyces its size is dependent on urine flow. The young infant frequently shows a prominent extrahilar pelvis which should not be mistaken for early hydronephrosis.

In the neonate and young infant the renal cortex is normally as echogenic as liver or spleen or even brighter. This feature may be explained by anatomical features peculiar to the neonate which increase the number of acoustic interfaces: (1) the glomeruli occupy proportionally a greater volume of the renal cortex during the first 2 months of life (18% as compared with 8.6% in the adult); (2) there is

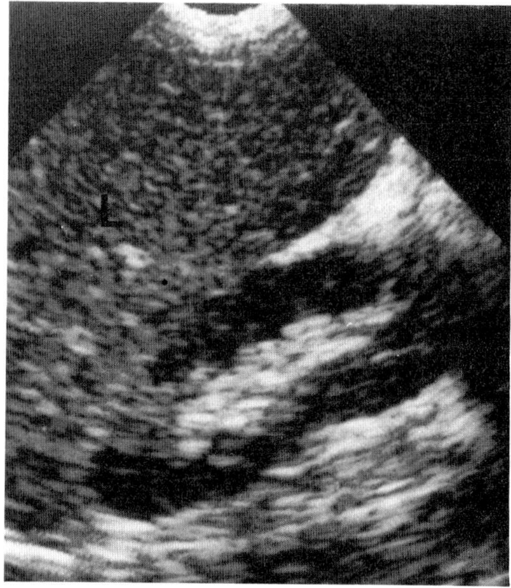

(a)

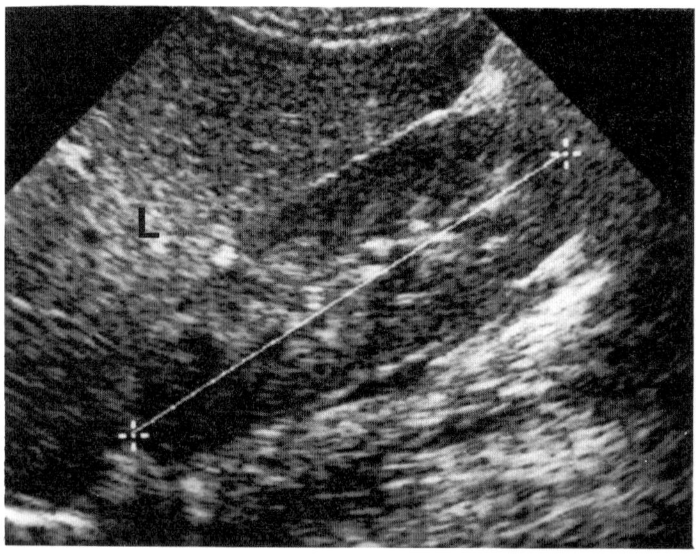

(b)

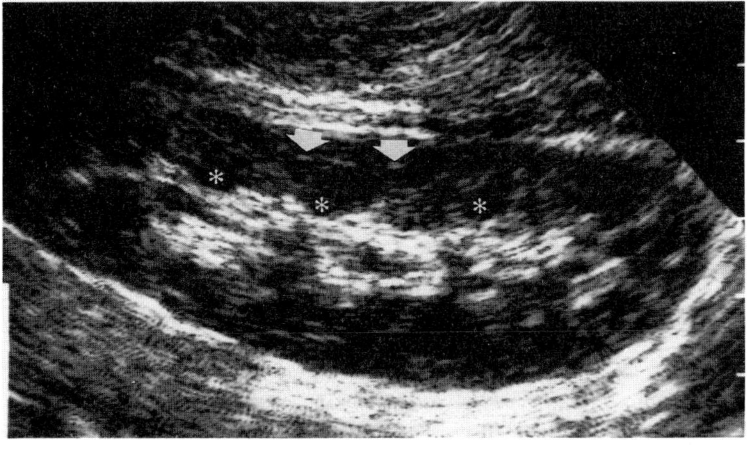

(c)

(d)

Figure 10.2 The normal kidney – longitudinal sections. (a) and (b) The right kidney in the supine position. The liver (L) has been used as an acoustic window. The central bright echoes are from the calyceal walls. Electronic calipers have been placed on the upper and lower poles of the kidney in (b) to measure bipolar length. (c) The left kidney viewed prone. The relatively echolucent papillae (*asterisks*) are seen adjacent to the bright calyceal walls and the arcuate arteries (*arrows*) mark the junction between cortex and medulla. (d) Prone view of the left kidney at the level of the renal hilum showing the bright echoes arising from the parapelvic fat (*curved arrows*)

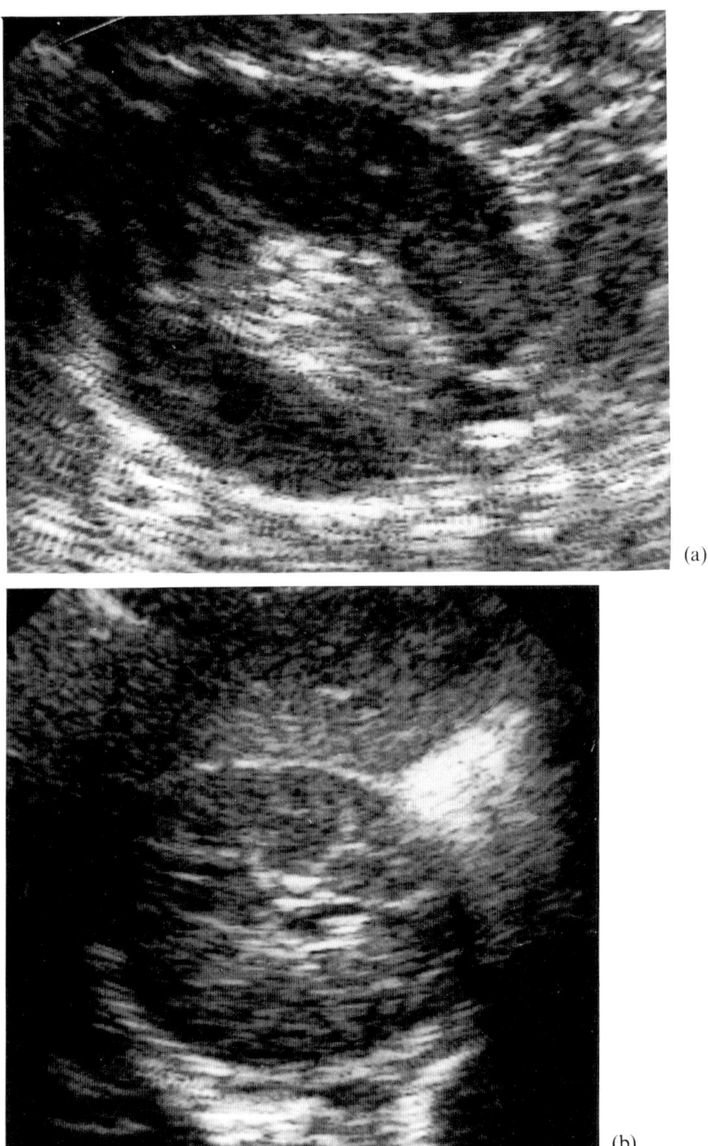

(a)

(b)

Figure 10.3 The normal kidney – transverse sections. (a) At the level of the renal hilum the bright echoes from parapelvic fat, vessel walls and pelvic wall give the kidney a horseshoe appearance. (b) Either side of the hilum the appearance is more like a doughnut with a central echo-free space due to urine in calyces surrounded by bright calyceal walls. (By convention, transverse scans of the abdomen and pelvis are displayed as if viewed from the bottom of the patient)

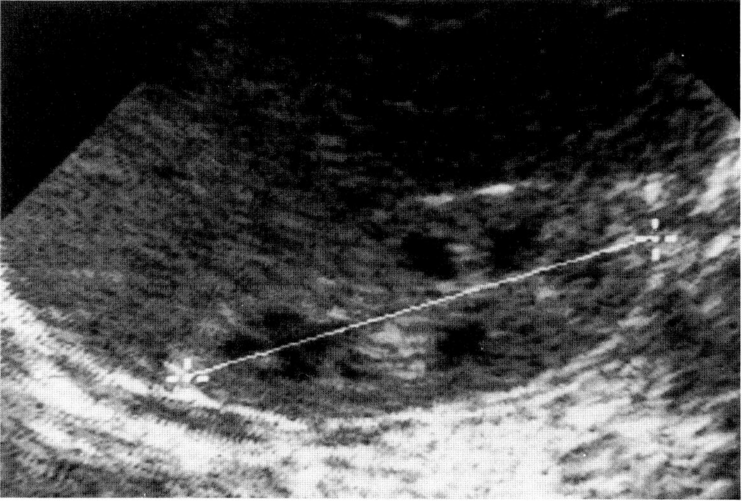

(a)

(b)

Figure 10.4 (a) and (b) Normal neonatal kidneys in longitudinal section. Cortical echogenicity is higher than (a) or similar to (b) liver. The prominent echolucent papillae should not be mistaken for dilated calyces. Cortical depressions (*arrows*) between renal pyramids are due to persistent fetal lobulation

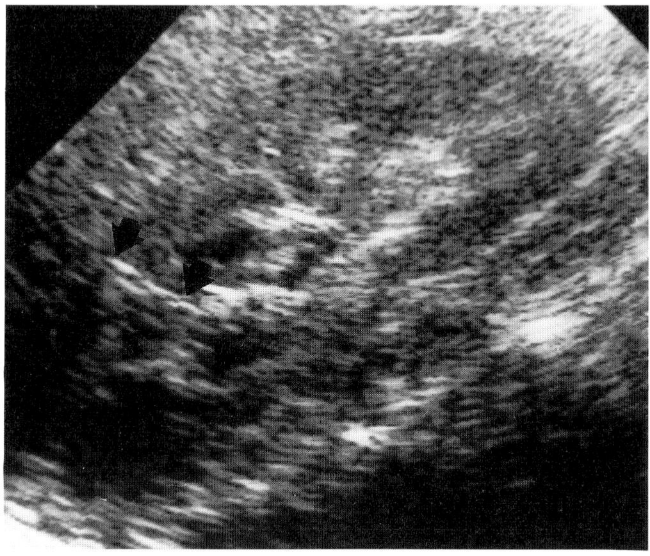

(a)

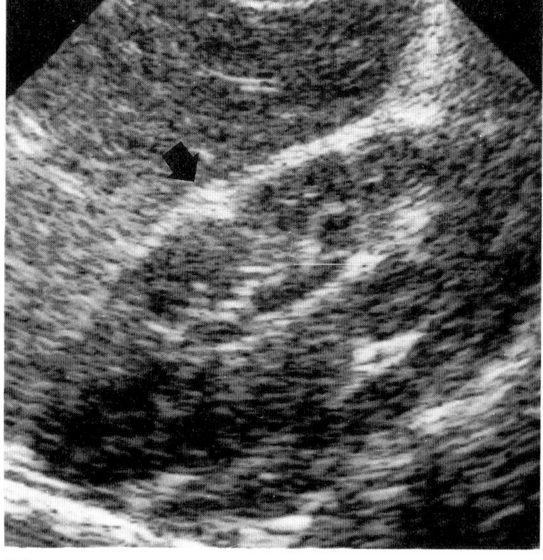

(b)

Figure 10.5 Parenchymal junctional line

a greater proportional volume in the cellular component of the glomerular tuft; and (3) 20% of the loops of Henle are located in cortex rather than the medulla (Hricak *et al.*, 1983). The very bright cortex makes the pyramids appear even more echolucent (Figure 10.4) and a failure to appreciate this feature at this age may lead to the mistaken diagnosis of hydronephrosis or multiple renal cysts. The echogenic renal cortex gradually progresses to the 'adult' appearance by 2–3 months of age but may occasionally persist until 6 months of age.

Increased echogenicity of renal pyramids in the newborn may be observed during treatment with frusemide, the mechanism probably being a transient hypercalciuria. Riebel and Wartner (1988) have shown transient increased echogenicity in the centre or tips of renal pyramids in neonates with normal renal function and believed the cause was mild Tamm–Horsfall proteinuria. Other features which distinguish the neonatal kidney from that of the older child are that the renal sinus region is less echogenic, presumably because there is less fat, and fetal lobulation is more frequently observed.

A common ultrasonic finding in the normal kidney is a thin echogenic linear structure running from the renal sinus to the cortex in an anterosuperior direction, the parenchymal junctional line (PJL) (Figure 10.5a). Superficially the PJL may appear as a small echogenic triangle or wedge on the anterior surface of the kidney (Figure 10.5b). In transverse section the PJL is seen to run anteriorly in the coronal plane. It is more frequently observed in the right kidney and should not be confused with a cortical scar (Kenney and Wild, 1987). The PJL is believed to originate from a layer of connective tissue which is trapped when a kidney is formed from the fusion of two metanephric elements.

Renal size

Measurement of renal length by US is easy to do but less reproducible than the radiographic method because it is difficult to scan knowingly along the longest axis of the kidney. A number of standards have been published which relate maximum renal length to age, weight, height, body surface area (Figure 10.6) and gestational age (Figure 10.7). It is also possible to calculate renal volume (Figure 10.8) using the formula:

$$V = L \times T \times W \times 0.5233$$

    where V = volume
           L = maximum length
           T = maximum thickness
           W = maximum width.

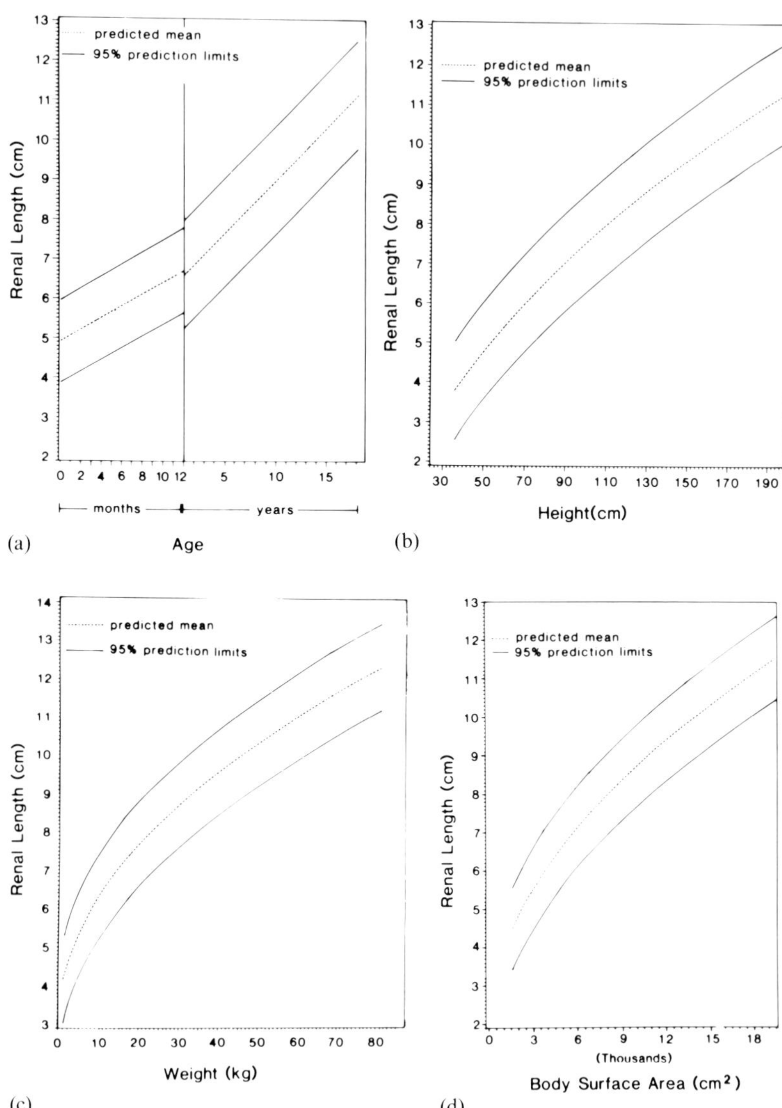

Figure 10.6 Bipolar renal length related to age (a), height (b), weight (c) and body surface area (d). (From Han and Babcock, 1985, by permission; © American Roentgen Ray Society, 1985)

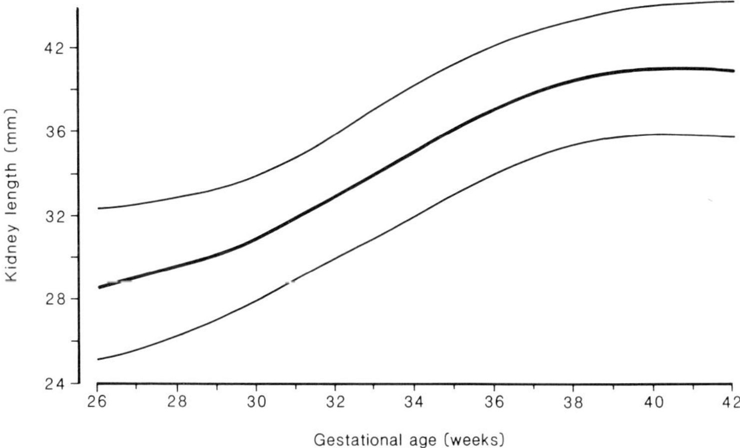

Figure 10.7 Bipolar renal length related to gestational age. (From DeVries and Levene, 1983, by permission of the authors and publishers)

Length measurements by US are not directly comparable with those obtained from EU as the latter are subject to geometric magnification, foreshortening caused by obliquity of the renal axis and swelling from the contrast medium-induced diuresis.

Ultrasonic patterns

Cystic (Figure 10.9)
Echo-free. Fluid causes very little attenuation of the sound beam and so the posterior wall of the cyst and the structures behind it are more echogenic than normal (posterior enhancement), e.g. bladder, renal pelvis, cyst, hydronephrosis, fresh haematoma.

Solid (Figure 10.10)
Low to high amplitude echoes without posterior enhancement, e.g. normal solid organs, tumour, organized haematoma.

Complex (Figure 10.11)
A mixture of echo-free and variable amplitude echoes, e.g. abscess, tumour, resolving haematoma, xanthogranulomatous pyelonephritis, complicated cyst (e.g. hydatid).

Shadows (Figure 10.12)
Very bright echoes with no echoes behind because all the sound has been reflected back to the transducer, e.g. calculi, calcification, bone.

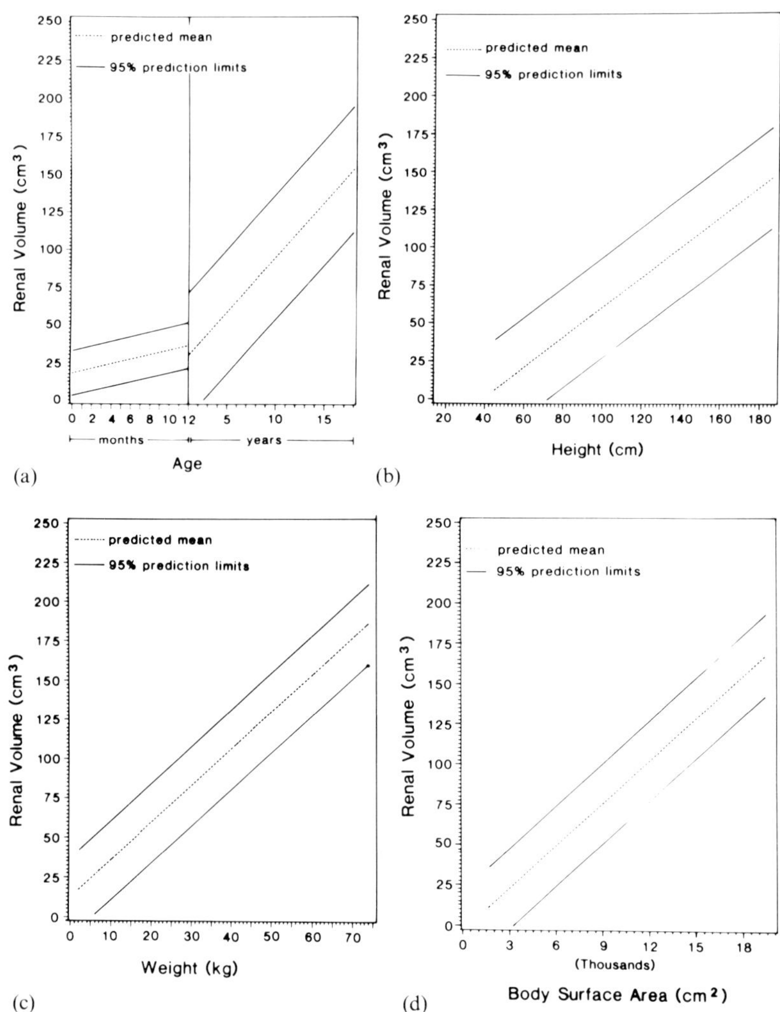

Figure 10.8 Renal volume related to age (a), height (b), weight (c) and body surface area (d). (From Han and Babcock, 1985, by permission; © American Roentgen Ray Society, 1985)

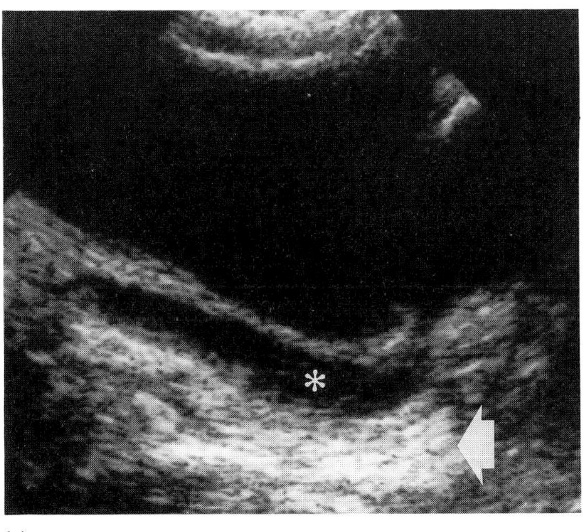

(a)

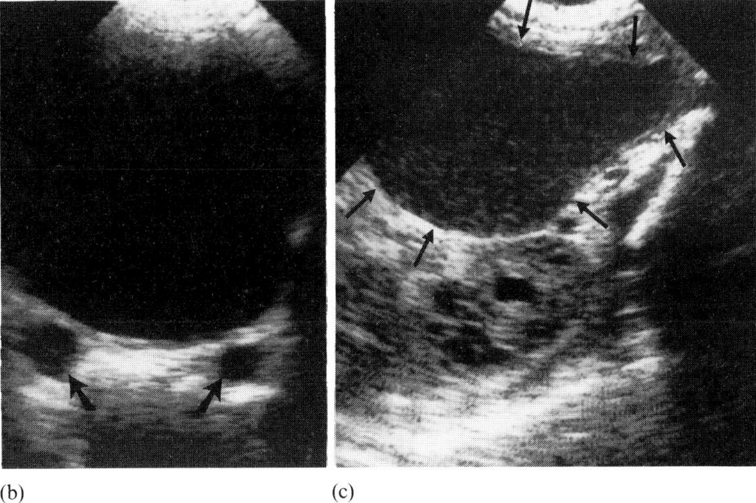

(b)   (c)

Figure 10.9 Examples of cystic structures as demonstrated by ultrasonography. (a) The bladder full of urine, seen here in longitudinal section. Fluid is typically echo free and because the sound beam is not attenuated by the fluid the echoes returning from structures behind it are brighter than usual (posterior enhancement, *arrow*). Dilated ureter (*asterisk*). (b) A full bladder seen in transverse section; both ureters (*arrows*) are dilated. (c) A longitudinal scan of the abdomen shows a large, fluid-filled structure (*arrows*), which on this occasion contains some echoes indicating that it is not clear fluid. This was, in fact, a hydrometrocolpos. A kidney is seen behind the cystic mass

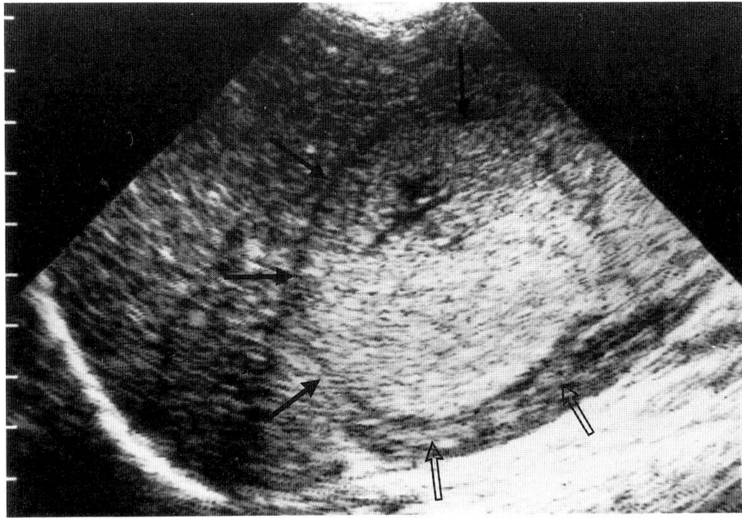

Figure 10.10 A solid mass – a Wilms' tumour (*black arrows*). In this longitudinal scan the tumour is seen to arise from the anterior surface of the right kidney (*white arrows*) which is flattened like a saucer posteriorly

Table 10.1   Causes of upper tract dilatation which may mimic obstruction

Normal variants

Scanning in the prone position	Mild calyceal separation is accentuated
Extrarenal renal pelvis	More common in the newborn
Full bladder	Confirmed by rescanning with the bladder empty
Diuresis	Overhydration or diuretics
Single kidney	
Congenital megacalyces	Rare

Renal cystic disease

Multicystic dysplastic kidney	No hilar cyst to be mistaken for a dilated renal pelvis. Cysts do not communicate
Adult-type polycystic disease	Calyces and pelvis are defined separate from the cysts

Inflammatory diseases

Reflux nephropathy	With loss of cortex which may show increased echogenicity
Tuberculosis	Cavity formation

Others

Vesico-ureteric reflux	
Atonia	Following relief of obstruction, prune belly syndrome
Papillary necrosis	Following sloughing of papillae

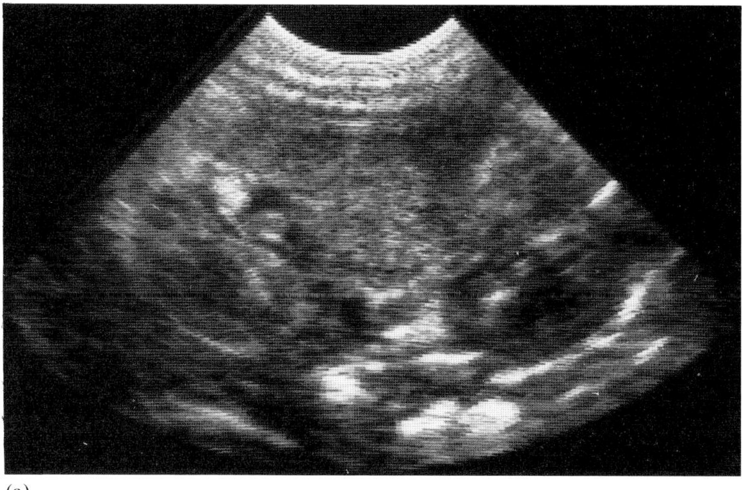

(a)

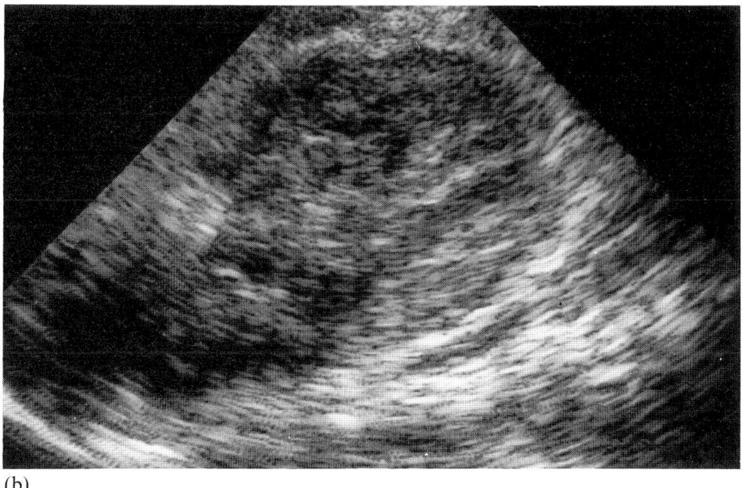

(b)

Figure 10.11 Complex echo patterns. (a) Renal vein thrombosis. (b) Renal trauma. Both kidneys show a disorganized echo pattern with foci of echolucency and echogenicity. The former is likely to be due to oedema and the latter to haematoma

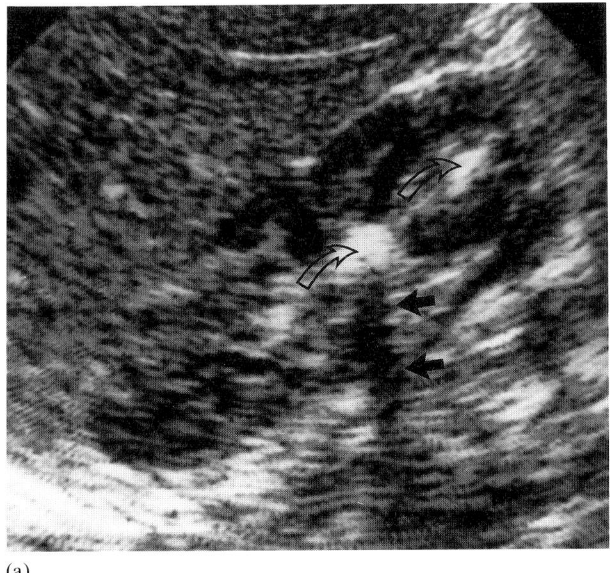

(a)

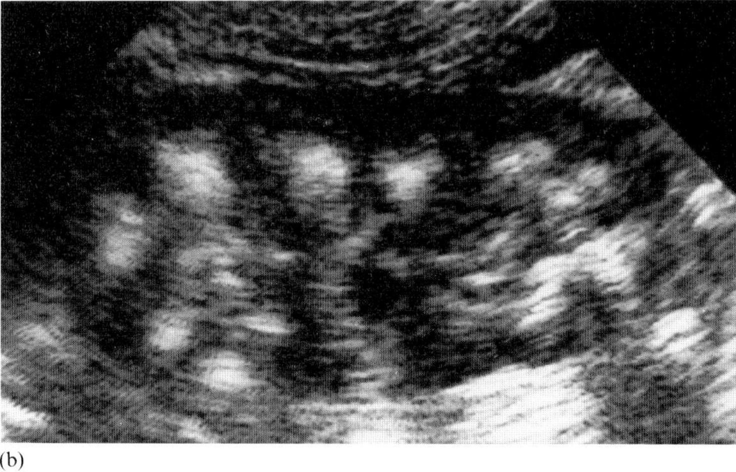

(b)

Figure 10.12 Bright echoes with posterior shadows are due to calcium or bone. (a) There are at least two calculi (*white arrows*) in this kidney. The largest lies in the middle of the kidney and exhibits prominent posterior shadowing (*black arrows*). (b) Echogenic renal papillae in a patient with nephrocalcinosis. Ultrasonography is more sensitive for nephrocalcinosis than plain abdominal radiography. (Figure A7.1a in Appendix 7 shows bright echoes with posterior shadowing due to ribs)

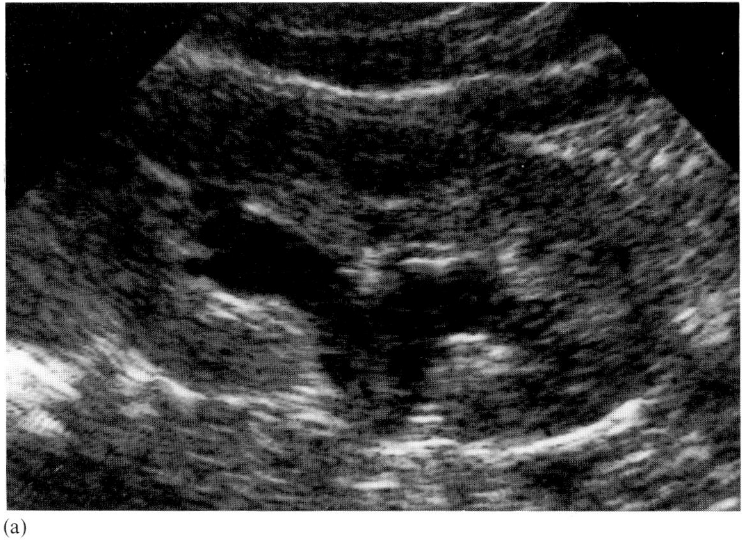

(a)

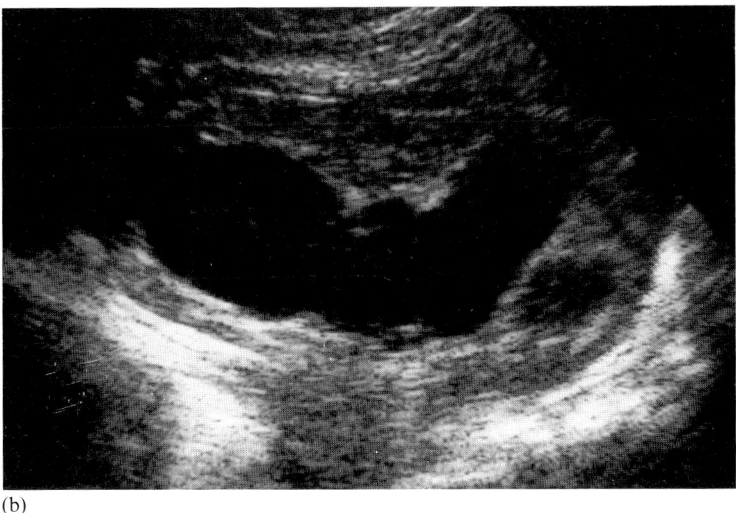

(b)

Figure 10.13 Hydronephrosis. (a) Compared with normal the bright central collection of echoes shows moderate separation due to urine within the calyces and pelvis. It is still easy to discern minor calyces arising from the upper pole major calyx. (b) More severe hydronephrosis.

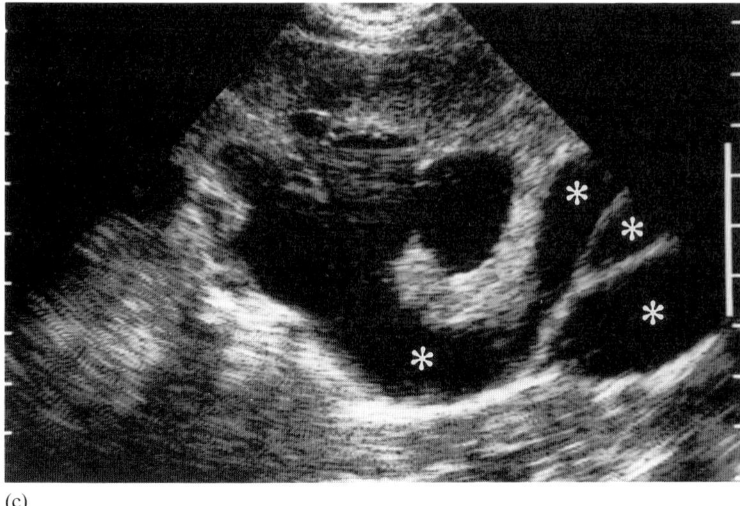

(c)

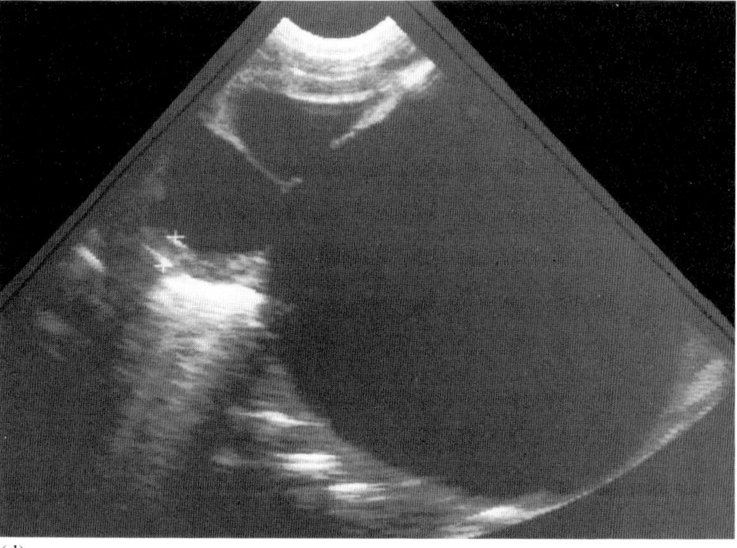

(d)

Figure 10.13 (*cont.*) (c) Hydronephrosis and a tortuous hydroureter (*asterisks*) clearly in continuity. (d) A hugely dilated renal pelvis is seen to communicate with dilated calyces. This demonstration of communication will exclude a multicystic kidney from the differential diagnosis and in the absence of a dilated ureter a pelvi-ureteric junction obstruction is most likely. The renal cortex, as described by the electronic calipers, is markedly thinned

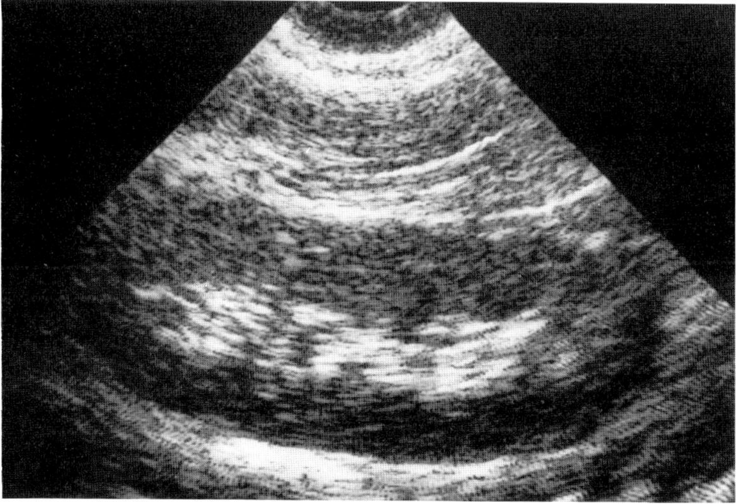

(a)

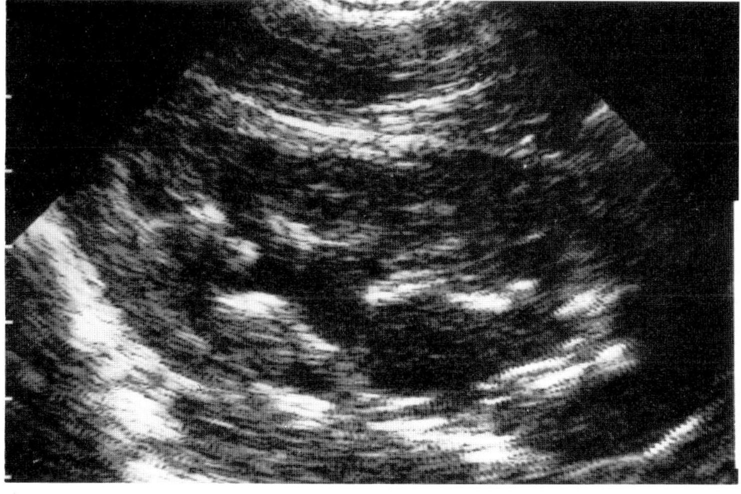

(b)

Figure 10.14 The value of a forced diuresis to diagnose a suspected pelvi-ureteric junction obstruction. A 12-year-old girl with recurrent right loin pain has a normal resting US. (a) Following provocation with i.v. frusemide the pelvis and calyces dilate and she experiences her usual pain (b)

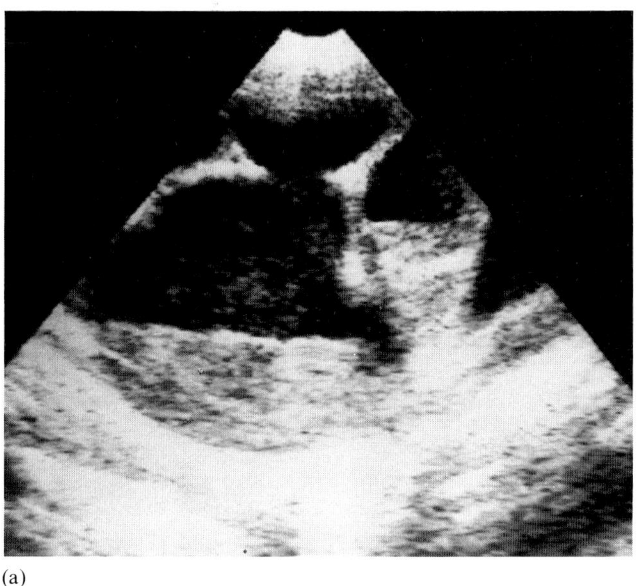

(a)

(b)

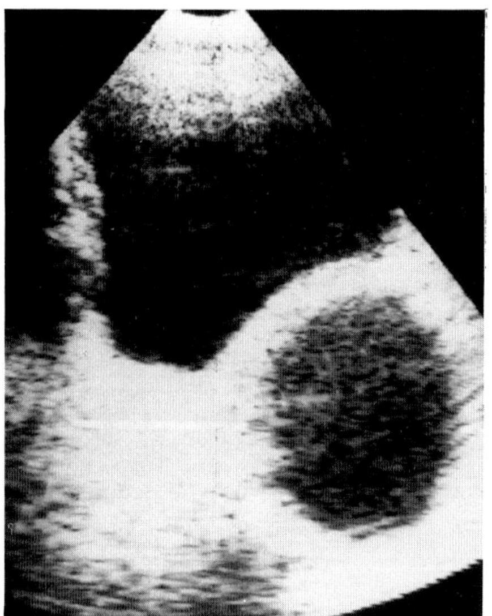

Figure 10.15 Pyonephrosis. (a) In longitudinal section the presence of multiple communicating cystic spaces indicates the presence of hydronephrosis, but in addition there are fluid levels within the calyces due to pus/urine interfaces.
(b) The transverse scan through the bladder indicates relatively echo-free urine within the bladder but the markedly dilated left ureter seen behind it contains numerous echoes indicative of pyuria and an obstruction at the ureterovesical junction.

Hydronephrosis

The US appearances of hydronephrosis are easily recognizable (Figure 10.13); a dilated cystic structure at the renal hilum represents a dilated pelvis and this communicates with other smaller cystic structures peripherally – the calyces. The sensitivity for diagnosing upper tract dilatation approaches 100% although not all cases will have a pathological cause (false-positive diagnoses) or be due to obstruction (Table 10.1). False-negative diagnoses include a staghorn calculus filling the pelvicalyceal system (but there will be acoustic shadowing), intermittent obstruction (a repeat examination following provocation with a diuresis is often useful; Figure 10.14), an incorrect diagnosis of cystic disease and misinterpretation of dilated calyces as prominent neonatal papillae. A pyonephrosis is suggested when urine within the dilated upper tract contains echoes and especially when a fluid level is demonstrable (Figure 10.15). It is important to determine the level of the obstruction by searching for ureteric dilatation, using the full bladder as an acoustic window (see Figure 10.9, p. 111).

Renal parenchymal disease

In the older infant and child with renal parenchymal disease the renal cortex becomes more echogenic than usual (Figure 10.16). Hricak *et al.* (1982) graded cortical echogenicity into four grades:

Grade 0:   Normal.
Grade I: Cortical echogenicity of the right kidney equals that of the liver.
Grade II: Cortical echogenicity of the right kidney is greater than that of the liver but less than that of the renal sinus.
Grade III: The echogenicity of the right renal cortex equals that of the renal sinus.

The intensity of cortical echogenicity correlates with the degree of parenchymal damage and represents global and/or segmental sclerosis of the glomeruli and/or interstitial changes such as fibrosis, tubular atrophy, interstitial infiltrate and deposition of calcium (Hayden and Swischuk, 1987). Ultrasonography is more sensitive than plain films for the detection of nephrocalcinosis and in the early stages of the disease the increased echoes from the calcium are not associated with acoustic shadowing. In the neonate US provides only an approximate guide to the severity of the disease process because cortical echogenicity is already high and renal sinus echoes are less prominent.

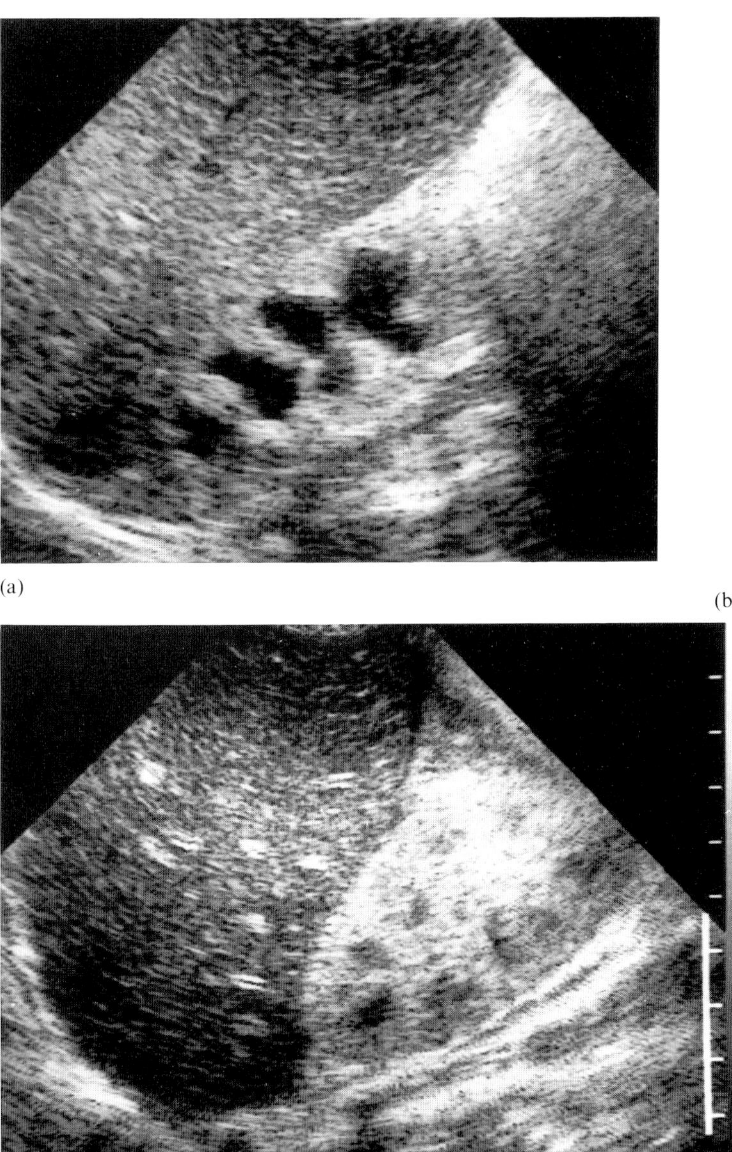

(a)

(b)

Figure 10.16 Increased cortical echogenicity relative to liver or spleen. (a) Thinned bright cortex with dilated calyces in a child with reflux nephropathy. (b) A swollen kidney with a bright cortex and echo-poor renal papillae, i.e. preserved cortico-medullary differentiation, in a child receiving induction chemotherapy for acute lymphoblastic leukaemia

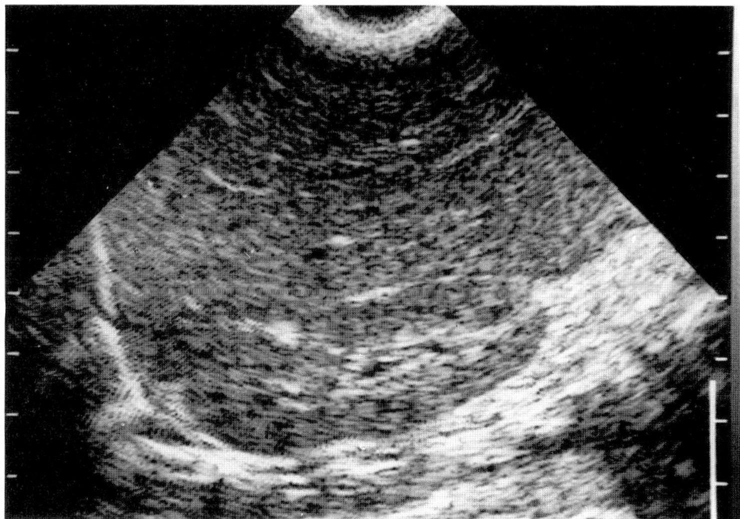

Figure 10.17 Increased parenchymal echogenicity with loss of corticomedullary differentiation

In general, there is poor correlation between the histological diagnosis and the sonographic appearance (Krensky, Reddish and Teele, 1983; Hayden *et al.*, 1984). Nevertheless it may be possible to narrow the diagnostic possibilities by considering renal size and noting the presence of cysts. Loss of corticomedullary differentiation (Figure 10.17) is considered by some to be helpful (Garel and Parente, 1986; Table 10.2) but does not reliably correlate with specific diagnoses. When it is lost significant parenchymal abnormality is present (Hayden *et al.*, 1984) but severe abnormality may be present when the corticomedullary junction is preserved.

Renal cystic disease

Ultrasonography is the imaging method *par excellence* for the detection of renal cysts. A useful classification of renal cystic disease is that provided by Elkin and Bernstein (1969) and simplified in Table 10.3.

The lower urinary tract

Normal anatomy

When the bladder is empty the entire pelvis is obscured by bowel gas. The bladder, filled with normal urine, is an echo-free cystic

Table 10.2   Correlation between kidney appearance on ultrasound with histological diagnosis (After Garel and Parente, 1986)

	Enlarged kidneys	Normal or only slight alteration of length	Small kidneys
Loss of CMD	Renal vein thrombosis* Infantile polycystic kidneys* (+ small macrocysts) Storage and infiltrative diseases* (e.g. acute lymphoblastic leukaemia)	Juvenile nephronophthisis (+ medullary cysts)*	End-stage disease* Dysplastic hypoplastic*
Reversed CMD	Juvenile polycystic kidneys (+ small macrocysts)	Medullary nephrocalcinosis Frusemide therapy in infants Transient phenomenon in newborns (? due to Tamm–Horsfall proteinuria)	
Preserved CMD	Renal vein thrombosis (early stage) Acute glomerulonephritis* Nephrotic syndrome* (except congenital Finnish type) Shock kidneys* Haemolytic uraemic syndrome*	Acute tubular necrosis Renal artery thrombosis Haemolytic uraemic syndrome*	Hypoplasia without dysplasia Oligomeganephronia*

*Indicates increased cortical echogenicity.
CMD: corticomedullary differentiation.

structure which is ovoid in longitudinal section and square in transverse section (Figure 10.21). The posterior wall of the bladder is indented, in the female, by the uterus. This organ is easy to identify at all ages but normal ovaries are elusive in the younger child. Lateral to the bladder are seen the ileopsoas muscles. The walls of the distended bladder are thin and smooth but when only partially filled they appear thickened with an irregular inner surface.

Using the urine-filled bladder as an acoustic window it is possible to visualize the extra- and intravesical parts of the ureter and to identify the submucosal ureteral segment (Marchal *et al.*, 1983). The exact site of the ureteric meatus may be located by observing the

Table 10.3   Classification of renal cystic disease

Renal dysplasia
   Multicystic dysplastic kidney (Figure 10.18)
   Focal and segmental cystic dysplasia
   Multiple cysts associated with lower urinary tract obstruction

Polycystic disease
   Infantile ⎫
   Juvenile ⎭ autosomal recessive (Figure 10.19)
   Adult   autosomal dominant (Figure 10.20)

Medullary cysts
   Medullary sponge kidney
   Juvenile nephronophthisis
   Calyceal cyst – essentially a calyceal diverticulum

Cortical cysts
   Simple cyst
   Tuberous sclerosis
   Trisomy 13 and 18
   Turner's syndrome
   Conradi's disease
   Zellweger syndrome
   Asphyxiating thoracic dystrophy

Neoplastic
   Benign cystic nephroma
   Cystic Wilms' tumour

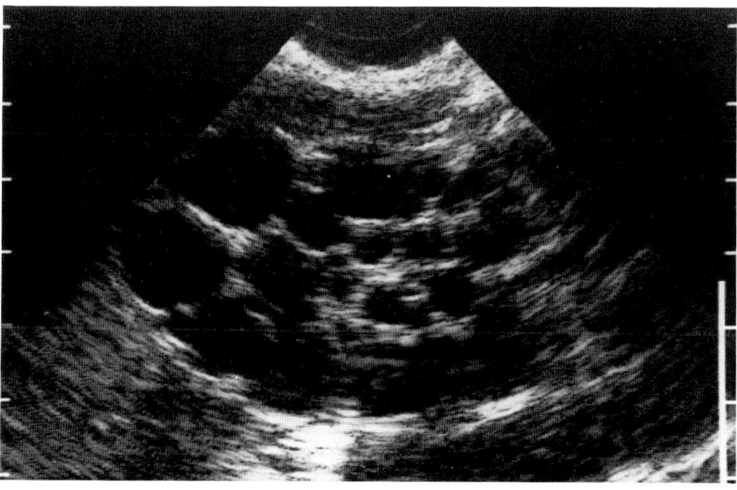

Figure 10.18 Multicystic kidney. Numerous small, discrete, non-communicating cysts

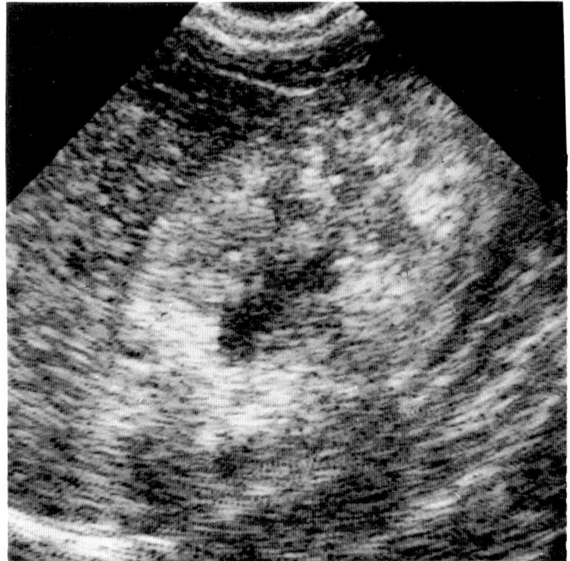

Figure 10.19 Recessive (infantile) polycystic renal disease

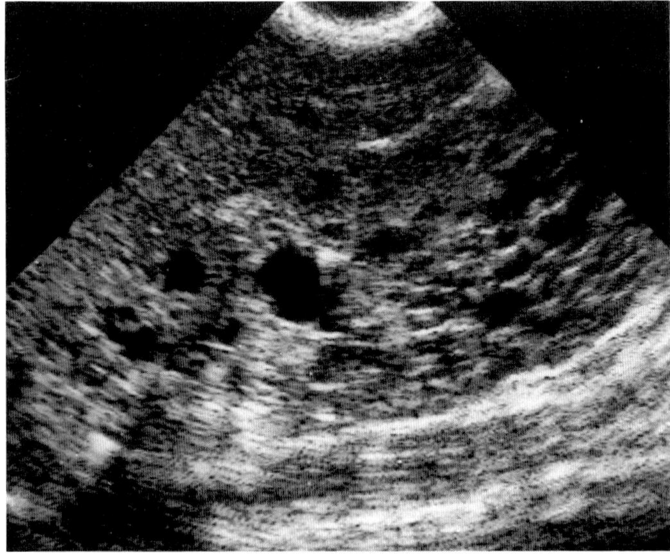

Figure 10.20 Dominant polycystic renal disease

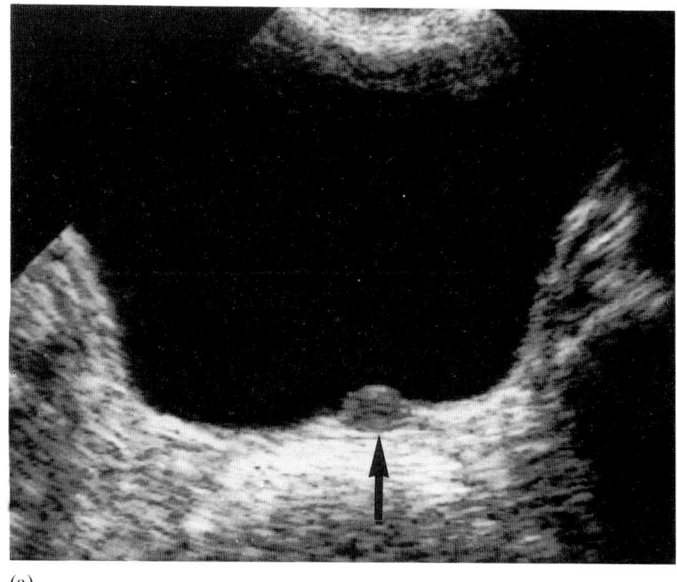

(a)

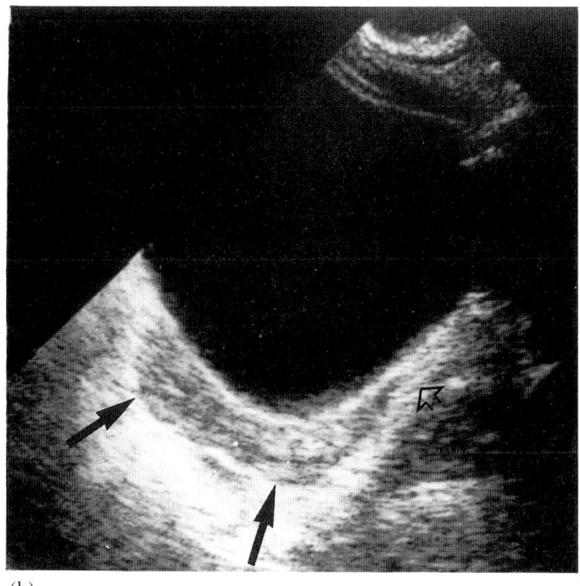

(b)

Figure 10.21 Normal bladder (a) in transverse and (b) in longitudinal section. Uterine body (*black arrows*). Uterine cervix (*white arrows*)

intermittent spurts of low-intensity echoes produced by the jet of urine entering the bladder (ureteric jet phenomenon).

References and further reading

Ultrasonography

Chopra, A. and Teele, R. L. (1980) Hydronephrosis in children: narrowing the differential diagnosis with ultrasound. *Journal of Clinical Ultrasound*, **8**, 473–478

Kangarloo, H., Gold, R. H., Fine, R. N. *et al.* (1985) Urinary tract infection in infants and children evaluated by ultrasound. *Radiology*, **154**, 367–373

Lebowitz, R. L. (1985) Paediatric uroradiology. *Pediatric Clinics of North America*, **32**, 1353–1362

Lebowitz, R. L. and Teele, R. L. (1983) Fetal and neonatal hydronephrosis. *Urologic Radiology*, **5**, 185–188

Leonidas, J. C., McCauley, R. G. K., Klauber, G. C. and Fretzayas, A. M. (1985) Sonography as a substitute for excretory urography in children with urinary tract infection. *American Journal of Roentgenology*, **144**, 815–819

Lindsell, D. and Moncrief, M. (1986) Comparison of ultrasound examination and intravenous urography after a urinary tract infection. *Archives of Disease in Childhood*, **61**, 81–82

Mason, Jr, W. G. (1984) Urinary tract infections in children: renal ultrasound evaluation. *Radiology*, **153**, 109–111

Miller, R. W., Fraumenti, J. F. and Manning, M. D. (1964) Association of Wilm's tumour with aniridia, hemihypertrophy and other congenital malformations. *New England Journal of Medicine*, **270**, 922–927

The upper urinary tract

DeVries, L. and Levene, M. I. (1983) Measurement of renal size in preterm and term infants by real-time ultrasound. *Archives of Disease in Childhood*, **58**, 145–147

Elkin, M. and Bernstein, J. (1969) Cystic diseases of the kidney – radiological and pathological considerations. *Clinical Radiology*, **20**, 65–82

Garel, L. and Parente, D. (1986) Ultrasound in paediatric nephrology. In *Paediatric Ultrasonography* (ed. G. Kalifa), Springer-Verlag, Berlin, pp. 173–188

Han, B. K. and Babcock, D. S. (1985) Sonographic measurements and appearance of normal kidneys in children. *American Journal of Roentgenology*, **145**, 611–616

Hayden, C. K., Jr and Swischuk, L. E. (1987) *Paediatric Ultrasonography*, Williams & Wilkins, Baltimore, p. 275

Hayden, C. K., Jr, Santa-Cruz, F. R., Amparo, E. G. *et al.* (1984) Ultrasonographic evaluation of the renal parenchyma in infancy and childhood. *Radiology*, **152**, 413–417

Hricak, H., Cruz, C., Romanski, R. *et al.* (1982) Renal parenchymal disease: sonographic-histologic correlation. *Radiology*, **144**, 141–147

Hricak, H., Slovis, T. L., Callen, C. W. *et al.* (1983) Neonatal kidneys: sonographic-anatomic correlation. *Radiology*, **147**, 699–702

Kenney, I. J. and Wild, S. R. (1987) The renal parenchymal junctional line in children: ultrasonic frequency and appearances. *British Journal of Radiology*, **60**, 865–868

Krensky, A. M., Reddish, J. M. and Teele, R. L. (1983) Causes of increased renal echogenicity in pediatric patients. *Pediatrics*, **72**, 840–846

Lebowitz, R. L. (1985) Paediatric uroradiology. *Pediatric Clinics of North America*, **32**, 1353–1362

Madewell, J. E., Hartman, D. S. and Lichtenstein, J. E. (1979) Radiologic-pathologic correlations in cystic disease of the kidney. *Radiologic Clinics of North America*, **17**, 261–279

Riebel, T. and Wartner, R. (1988) Ultrasonographic detection of uncommon hyperechogenic structures in kidneys among neonates and young babies. In *Proceedings of the 25th Congress of the European Society Paediatric Radiology* (Montreux, 1988)

The lower urinary tract

Marchal, G. J., Baert, A. L., Eeckels, R. and Proesmans, W. (1983) Sonographic evaluation of the normal ureteral submucosal tunnel in infancy and childhood. *Paediatric Radiology*, **13**, 125–129

Chapter 11

Imaging: nuclear medicine

Radionuclide renal imaging is widely used in the diagnosis and follow-up of paediatric renal disease. The low radiation dose coupled with the absence of systemic side-effects has led to a rapid expansion in its use. Depending on the type of study employed it may be used to assess renal perfusion, function and drainage. In the neonate there is rarely an indication to perform excretion urography (EU) as the kidneys are only poorly visualized because of the low glomerular filtration rate (GFR). Excretion urography, particularly in this age-group, may be misleading and ultrasonography with or without radionuclide imaging usually provides the correct diagnosis. Radionuclide studies do, however, fail to provide the detailed anatomical information provided by other imaging modalities.

^{99m}Technetium emits pure gamma rays with an energy of 140 keV and is an ideal isotope for imaging with a gamma camera. It can be labelled to a variety of different compounds to produce different radiopharmaceuticals which allow the imaging of different organs and cell series. The energy detected by the gamma camera is processed and analysed by a dedicated computer.

Radiopharmaceuticals

^{99m}Technetium DTPA

^{99m}Technetium (Tc) is a widely available radionuclide with a short half-life (6 hours) and the energy of its gamma ray emissions (140 keV) is ideally suited to gamma camera imaging. Ninety-five per cent of the administered dose of ^{99m}Tc-diethylenetriamine pentacetic acid (Tc-DTPA) is cleared by glomerular filtration with no significant tubular excretion or renal retention. The rate of clearance gives an accurate estimate of GFR (see Chapter 5). Dynamic imaging of the kidneys, ureters and bladder can be performed but because of its low retention in the renal cortex static imaging is not possible and small cortical lesions will not be demonstrated.

Dose
Adult, 75 MBq; child, 1 MBq kg^{-1} (minimum 4 MBq).

^{99m}Technetium DMSA

^{99m}Technetium dimercaptosuccinic acid (Tc-DMSA) is 90% bound to plasma proteins with only a small fraction passing through the glomerulus into the urine. It is incorporated principally into the proximal convoluted tubules directly from the blood by being bound to soluble cytoplasmic proteins and mitochondria, and to a lesser extent to microsomes and nuclei. The images obtained are of functioning tubular mass.

Dose
Adult, 75 MBq; child, 3.7 MBq kg^{-1}.

^{99m}Technetium glucoheptonate

Like Tc-DTPA this is rapidly cleared from the blood but, unlike Tc-DTPA, by a combination of both glomerular filtration and tubular uptake. Excellent dynamic images are possible and with approximately 20% of the dose being retained in the tubular cells images of the renal cortex can be obtained by delayed imaging at 2–4 hours. Static image quality is, however, inferior to that obtained with Tc-DMSA, particularly in the presence of renal failure. Because of the dual route of excretion GFR cannot be measured with this radiopharmaceutical.

^{123}Iodine orthoiodohippurate

^{123}Iodine is a cyclotron-produced isotope which limits its widespread availability. It is cleared from the blood in a similar way to para-aminohippuric acid, i.e. by a combination of glomerular filtration (20%) and tubular secretion (80%) and the rate of clearance equates with effective renal plasma flow (ERPF).

Dose
Adult, 12 MBq; child, 0.2 MBq kg^{-1} (minimum 3 MBq).

Radiographic contrast media and radiopharmaceuticals

Contrast media used in urography and arteriography have a temporary deleterious effect on the uptake and transit of radiopharmaceuticals used in renal imaging. Radionuclide studies should be performed before or 48 hours after the administration of contrast medium (Treves *et al.*, 1985).

Dynamic imaging: renography

Renography records the arrival, uptake, transit and excretion of a radiopharmaceutical by the kidneys following its intravenous injection. The radiopharmaceutical of current choice is ^{99m}Tc-DTPA.

Indications for a DTPA scan

1. To differentiate obstructive from non-obstructive dilatation of the urinary tract. This follows from information already obtained from ultrasonography or excretion urography and is answered by diuretic renography.
2. To assess relative renal function. When one kidney contributes over 15% of total renal function it should be conserved, but if it contributes less than 7% of total function restoration of significant function is usually not possible. When combined with estimation of GFR it is a simple matter to estimate individual kidney GFR.
3. To assess renal perfusion following renal transplantation and trauma.

Technique

To obtain consistent results all patients must be maintained in an adequate state of hydration during the examination. Babies must not miss a feed and infants and older children should be given a drink on arrival in the nuclear medicine department. Dehydration will result in sluggish urine flow and an obstructive pattern will be mimicked. Thus it is unwise to perform renography on the same day as excretion urography as the patient may be dehydrated for the latter investigation. If possible the patient empties the bladder prior to the examination and either sits with his or her back to the gamma camera or lies on it in the case of the younger child. Renal transplant recipients also lie supine but with the camera positioned at the front. The examination may last up to 30 minutes during which time the child must be perfectly still. Appropriate sedation will be necessary for the less cooperative child. A crying, moving child will result in inaccurate information from regions of interest (see below) and movement, particularly in the first 3 minutes, may produce erroneous results leading to the wrong decision regarding nephrectomy or conservation. The patient is positioned so that the camera covers both kidneys and bladder.

The appropriate dose of radiopharmaceutical is administered as a rapid intravenous bolus through a 23G or 25G butterfly and followed with a saline flush. The injection is made with the patient's arm abducted away from the gamma camera so that activity within the arm is not counted by the computer. The butterfly should be left in the vein if the administration of a diuretic is anticipated. For the sedated child a cannula should be inserted prior to, or at the same time as, the administration of a sedative so that the child will not be disturbed by the venepuncture. Thirty-second frames are stored by a computer for 20–30 min and analogue images obtained every 5 min. The study is monitored on a persistence oscilloscope and if there is no retention of radiopharmaceutical to suggest obstruction then no diuretic is given and the study is terminated at 20 min. If a diuretic renogram is indicated (see below) the diuretic is administered at 20 min and the study continued until there is obvious washout of activity from the kidneys or for a further 10–15 min, whichever is sooner.

If this standard procedure is not to be followed by indirect radionuclide cystography (see below) the child should empty the bladder to reduce the radiation dose to the bladder wall.

Computer analysis and interpretation

Regions of interest are drawn for both kidneys, bladder and tissue/blood background (Figure 11.1). In certain situations it may be necessary to draw special regions of interest, e.g. around each of the moieties of a duplex kidney or renal parenchyma and renal pelvis. Curves of count rates v. time are generated by the computer for each region and corrected for background activity.

The results of the investigation are presented as a series of analogue images (Figure 11.2), computer-processed digital images (Figure 11.3) and a set of background subtracted curves (Figure 11.4). The images are a summation of activity at timed intervals after the injection of radiopharmaceutical. Calyces are only poorly visualized but the renal pelvis is seen at 4–5 min. The bladder appears at 5–10 min and activity rises steadily as the kidneys drain. The renogram curves display count rate against time for each region of interest. The kidney curves show three classic phases.

First phase
This is a rapid rise in activity a few seconds after the intravenous

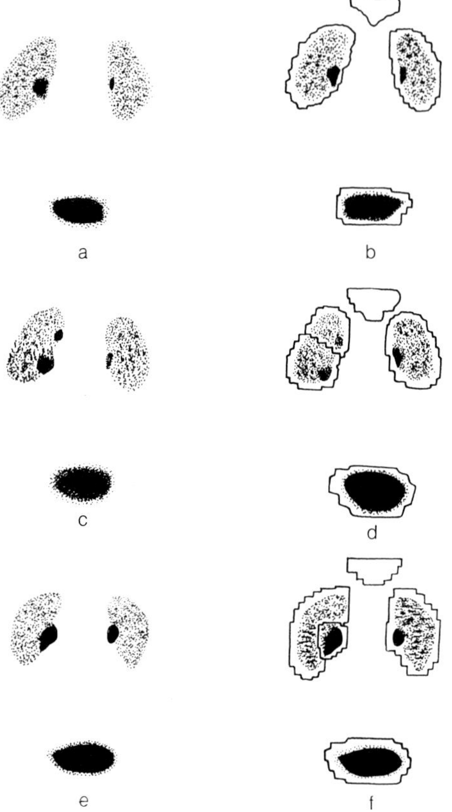

Figure 11.1 Regions of interest drawn on summed images. (a) and (b) Both kidneys, bladder and background. (c) and (d) Separate regions of interest for each moiety of a duplex kidney. (e) and (f) Separate regions of interest for parenchyma and pelvis

injection and is a reflection not only of the vascular supply to the kidney but also of the speed of the injection.

Second phase

After a few seconds the rapid rise is replaced by a more gradual slope which reflects renal handling of isotope as it is taken up by kidney and passes down the nephrons. The curve rises because at this particular time more isotope is being extracted by the kidney than is leaving it by excretion. The second phase reaches a peak at 2–5 min (the time to peak), at which time about 5% of the injected dose is in

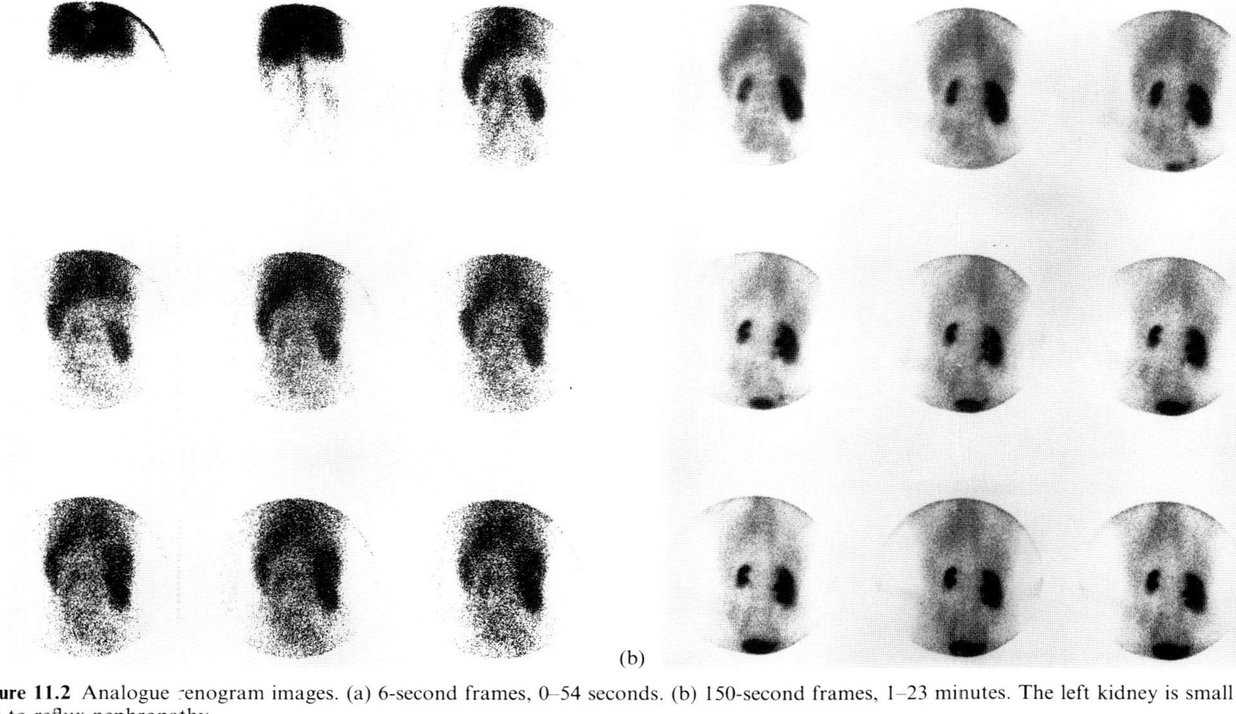

(a)

(b)

Figure 11.2 Analogue renogram images. (a) 6-second frames, 0–54 seconds. (b) 150-second frames, 1–23 minutes. The left kidney is small due to reflux nephropathy

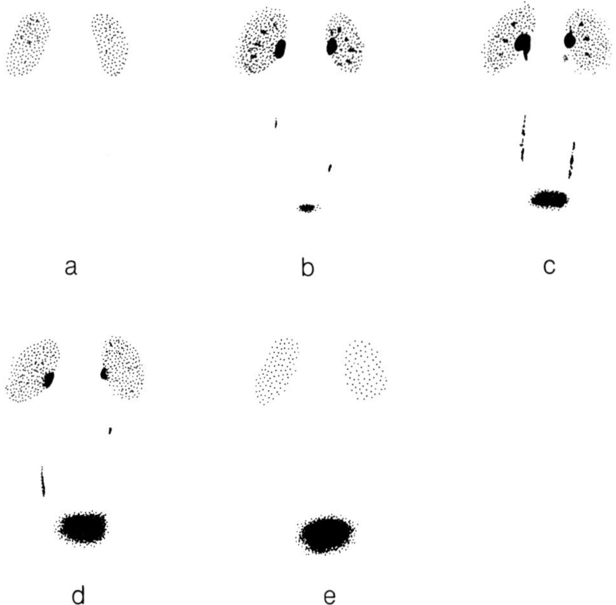

Figure 11.3 Diagrammatic representation of computer-processed summed renogram images. (a) 0–2½ minutes. (b) 2½–5 minutes. (c) 5–10 minutes. (d) 10–15 minutes. (e) 15–20 minutes

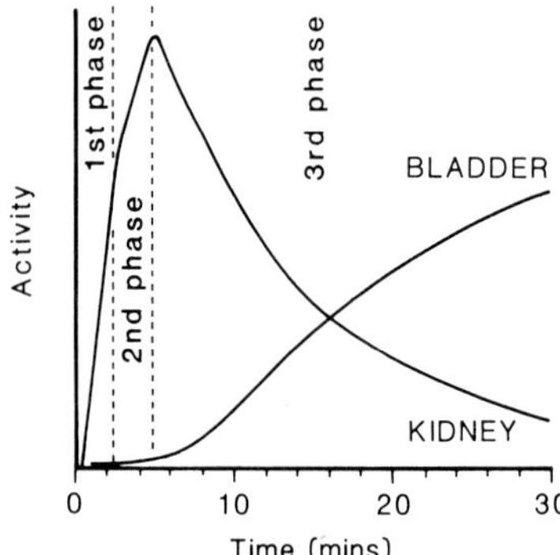

Figure 11.4 Renogram. Background subtracted curves

each kidney. A delayed time to peak is seen in a number of conditions including obstruction (prevention of excretion), renal artery stenosis (more prolonged arrival of isotope), low urine flow rate and parenchymal disease (O'Reilly, Shields and Testa, 1987).

Third phase
Following the peak the curve descends reflecting the situation of excretion outweighing extraction. The onset of the third phase coincides with the first appearance of activity within the bladder. This phase is highly sensitive to abnormalities of the outflow tract and a normal curve excludes even trivial obstruction.

Occasionally the normal third phase may descend in a stepwise manner (Figure 11.5), which may represent a variation in the volume and speed of bolus formation and peristaltic rate (O'Reilly, Shields and Testa, 1987). Sawtooth waves (Figure 11.6) may also be observed. When gross they may be indicative of vesico-ureteric reflux; minor degrees can be seen in the obstructed ureter and are due to retrograde peristaltic waves.

If a kidney is non-functioning the unsubtracted renogram curve

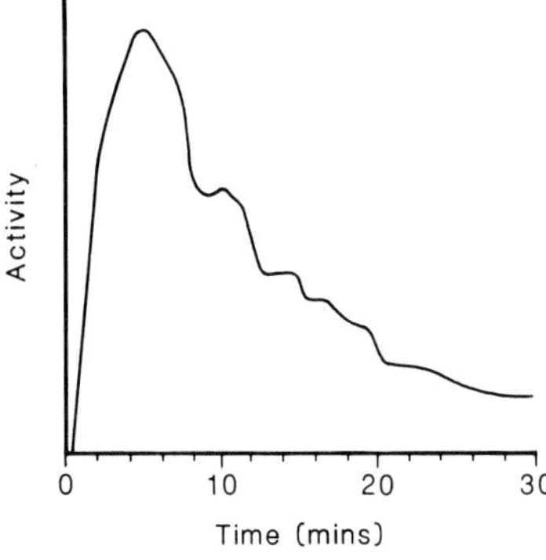

Figure 11.5 Renogram. Stepwise third phase

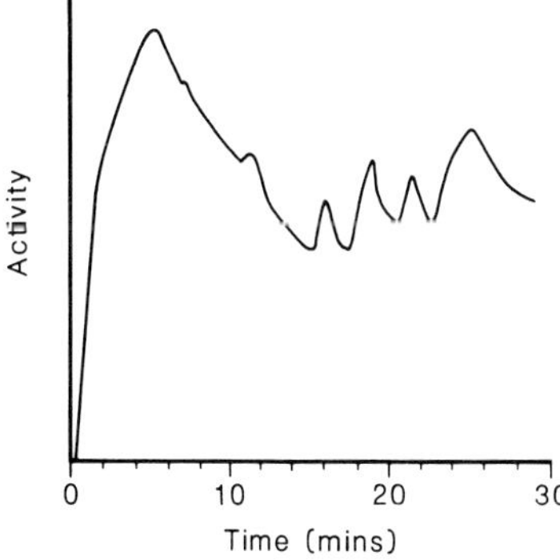

Figure 11.6 Renogram. Sawtooth third phase

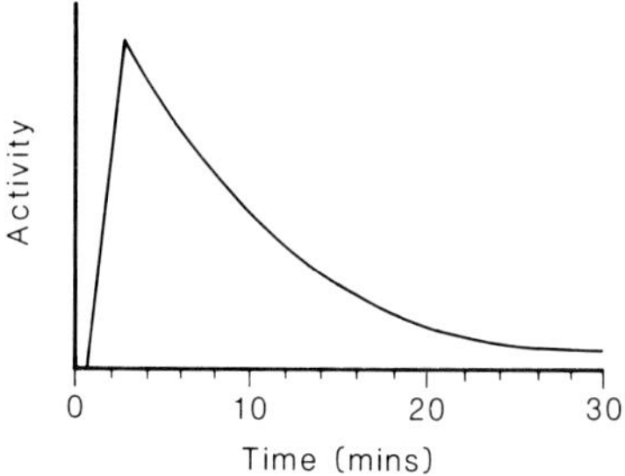

Figure 11.7 Unsubtracted renogram curve of a non-functioning kidney; identical to blood background. The blood background subtracted curve would be completely flat

will be identical to the blood background curve and the background subtracted curve will be flat (Figure 11.7).

Differential renal function

Differential or relative renal function can be calculated from the renal activity recorded between the first 80 and 180 s, i.e. the second phase, of the scan before there is significant activity in the collecting systems. During this time all the activity within the kidney is due to perfused renal tissue and activity in renal tubules. Assuming both kidneys are equidistant from the gamma camera, then during the second phase the ratio of background-corrected activity for each kidney will be equal to the ratio of their GFRs (if DTPA is used) or ERPFs (if OIH is used). Orthoiodohippurate will produce more accurate results and clearer pictures with reduced renal function because renal extraction of hippuran is four times more efficient than DTPA and thus the target-to-background ratio is much improved (Jewkes and Jayasingh, 1981). However, even with OIH, dynamic renal scans are of little use when the serum creatinine is above $500\,\mu\text{mol}\,1^{-1}$.

It is important to realize that if one kidney has markedly decreased or delayed function then by the time that kidney had accumulated enough activity for analysis there will be such a large amount of activity in the collecting system of the contralateral kidney that a valid comparison between the two kidneys is impossible.

The neonate

Both glomerular and tubular function are reduced in the newborn and immature glomerular function severely limits the value of EU at this time, making radionuclide studies particularly useful. The results of DTPA studies are, however, also less good in the first few days of life and show reduced uptake of radionuclide, poor kidney-to-background ratios and prolonged intrarenal transit and excretion. Glomerular function improves rapidly in the first 96 hours of life and then increases slowly to adult levels by the age of 3 years.

Hydronephrosis and diuresis renography

On the early analogue images the hydronephrotic kidney appears as a photon-deficient area, the size of which depends on the size of the dilated pelvicalyceal system. This is surrounded by a rim of activity in the renal parenchyma. Later images show accumulation of isotope in the dilated pelvis and calyces. The time activity curve reflects the changes evident on the analogue images (Figure 11.8). As the degree of dilatation increases the third phase becomes straight, then convex upwards. The time to peak is delayed and finally in complete obstruction no peak occurs and the second phase persists. Retention of isotope within the kidney may, however, be due to other causes, in particular dehydration and dilatation without obstruction. Problems related to dehydration will be negated by good technique; the diuretic renogram was introduced to differentiate true obstruction from dilatation without obstruction (O'Reilly *et al.*, 1978).

At low flow rates the non-obstructed, dilated urinary tract will appear obstructed because of stasis of isotope but at the high flow

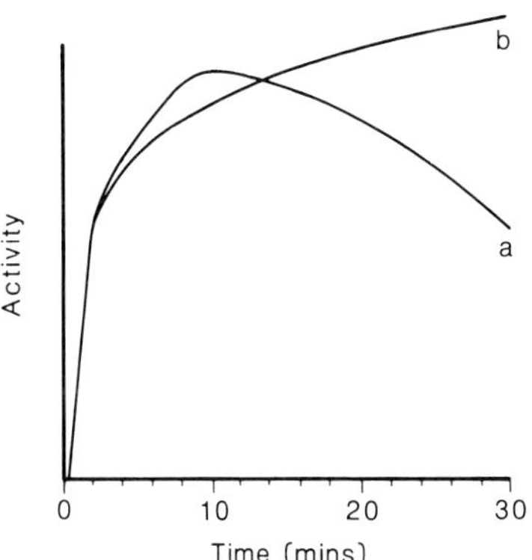

Figure 11.8 Renogram in obstruction. (a) Early obstruction with elevation and convexity of the third phase. (b) Severe obstruction with impaired uptake and a rising third phase

rate initiated by a diuretic the isotope will be washed out. The truly obstructed urinary tract will be obstructed at both low and high flow rates. The technique is now described.

The initial part of the study is as for the conventional renogram described above. The child must be well hydrated to ensure a good response to the diuretic. At 20 min frusemide 0.5 mg kg^{-1} is given intravenously and images are acquired for a further 10–20 min. It is possible to give the diuretic prior to the radiopharmaceutical but with that method it is not possible to compare before and after curves, which is often most helpful. Caution should be exercised

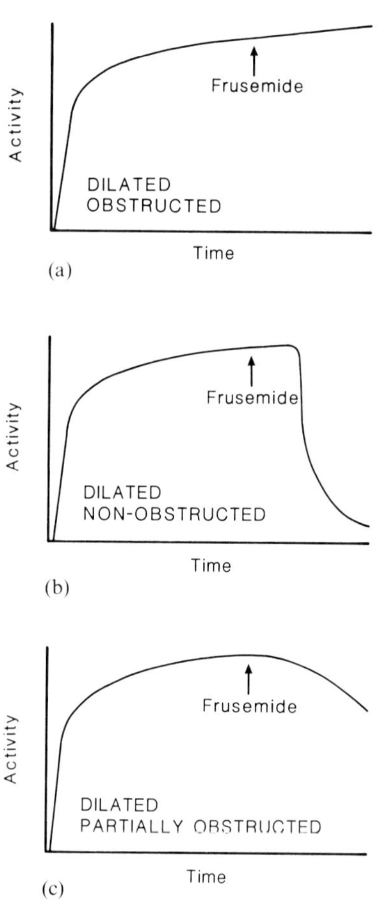

Figure 11.9 The obstructed renogram curve and response to frusemide. (a) Dilated and obstructed. (b) Dilated but not obstructed. (c) Dilated and partially obstructed

when interpreting the response to frusemide when renal function is severely impaired, when the system is grossly dilated or when the bladder is overdistended. In the latter situation repeat images should be obtained following micturition or bladder catheterization and drainage. The differing responses of the dilated upper urinary tract to the administration of frusemide are illustrated in Figure 11.9. Those children with equivocal results may need more invasive methods of investigation such as the Whitaker test.

Those patients who experience loin pain because of intermittent hydronephrosis due to incomplete obstruction may have their pain reproduced when high urine flow produces overdistension of a renal pelvis.

It is possible to investigate a dilated ureter by this method. The region of interest must be placed just proximal to the suspected site of obstruction and not over the kidney as the renogram curve for the latter may show adequate drainage when the urine drains into the capacious but dilated ureter (O'Reilly, 1986).

Deconvolution of the renogram

The radiopharmaceutical is not completely cleared from the blood immediately after injection and extraction continues for the duration of the examination at a rate proportional to its concentration and the GFR. Thus the standard renogram curves represent the response of the kidney to a changing concentration of isotope, which rises rapidly initially and then falls gradually during the examination. Deconvolution is a mathematical technique which aims to illustrate the effect of a single instantaneous bolus of radiopharmaceutical injected into the renal arteries and without recirculation. A normal deconvoluted renogram curve is illustrated in Figure 11.10. This is also given the term 'impulse retention function' or 'unit impulse response' (UIR) – the response of a kidney to an impulse of activity.

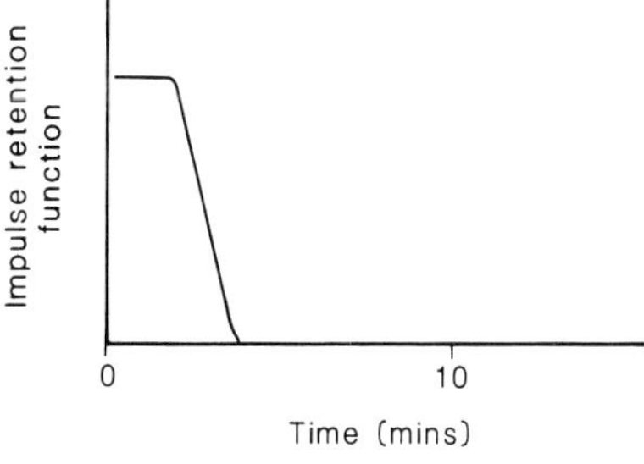

Figure 11.10 Deconvoluted renogram curve

The first part of the curve is a plateau, which represents the isotope which has entered the kidney. The length of this plateau indicates the shortest transit time of isotope through the kidney while the time taken for the curve to fall to zero is the longest transit time. The slope of the curve between shortest and longest times is the spread of transit times and the mean whole kidney transit time (WKTT) is frequently quoted in renogram results and is normally 2–3 min. Like the conventional renogram curve prolongation of WKTT does not distinguish between the obstructed dilated pelvis and the unobstructed dilated pelvis. The relative initial heights of the plateaus of each kidney are proportional to their relative GFRs.

A further modification of technique that is useful in evaluating the hydronephrotic kidney is to compare WKTT with mean parenchymal transit time (MPTT). In the presence of significant renal outflow obstruction salt and water reabsorption in the proximal tubule is increased and both WKTT and MPTT are prolonged. When the renal pelvis is dilated but not obstructed WKTT is prolonged but MPTT is normal. A satisfactory improvement in renal function following relief of obstruction is more likely when MPTT is normal than if it is prolonged. Regions of interest are drawn around the whole kidney, the renal parenchyma, excluding the renal pelvis, and a region for background subtraction (see Figure 11.1f). This technique has a 80% correlation with diuretic renography but in small children results should be interpreted with care as it may not be easy to separate the thin renal parenchyma from the pelvis on the small renal images of infants.

Static renal imaging

The principal radiopharmaceutical used for static imaging is Tc-DMSA. Tc-glucoheptonate is less widely employed and [67]gallium citrate and [111]indium-labelled white cells are of limited use in inflammatory renal disease.

Indications for Tc-DMSA scan

1. Assessment of differential renal function, especially when a decision is to be made as to whether a kidney is worth conserving or nephrectomy is indicated. In the presence of obstruction or infection it is not possible to assess the extent of recoverability that may be possible, but when one kidney contributes less than 7% of total renal function recovery usually fails. Relative function of the two moieties of a duplex kidney is also possible

(Figure 11.11). The radiation dose to the kidney is approximately 15 times higher with DMSA than with DTPA but DMSA has the advantage of a higher kidney-to-background ratio in the presence of moderate or severe renal failure. The limit of normal differential function is 45%:55%.

2. Assessment of non-functioning cortical tissue, in particular renal scars. A normal scan (posterior and both posterior oblique projections) excludes focal renal parenchymal pathology (Merrick, Utley and Wild, 1980). Acute pyelonephritis will result in a temporary impairment of renal activity and the assessment of long-term damage, i.e. scarring, should wait 2 months after antibiotic therapy.

3. In a girl with diurnal enuresis in whom an ectopic ureter is suspected US of the kidney may be normal if the upper moiety of a duplex kidney is dysplastic rather than hydronephrotic. A Tc-DMSA scan may detect an occult upper moiety (Figure 11.11).

4. Assessment of function in normal renal tissue, e.g. a hypertrophied septum of Bertin and the isthmus of a horseshoe kidney.

5. To determine the presence and position of an ectopic kidney. Anterior views must be obtained when activity is seen in only one kidney on the posterior projection.

6. Renovascular hypertension. Foci of decreased activity correlate

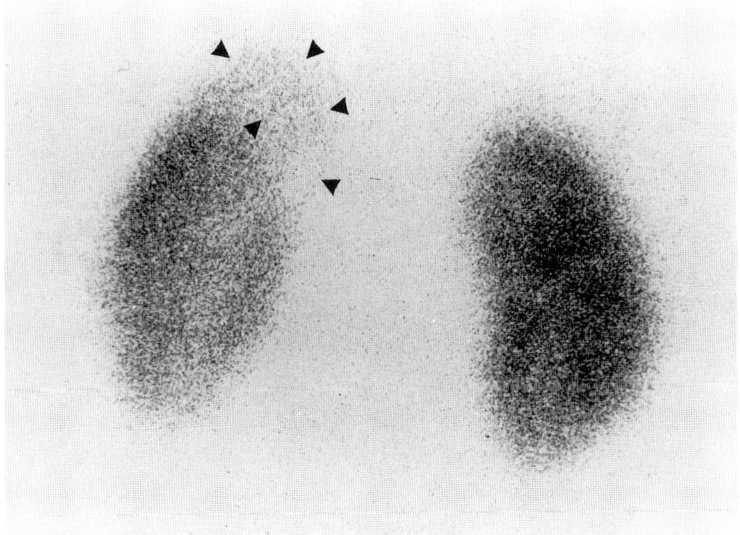

Figure 11.11 Tc-DMSA scan showing poor function in the upper pole of a left duplex kidney. The right kidney is normal

with ischaemic tissue and areas affected by vasculitis. A normal scan excludes most renovascular causes of hypertension with the exception of main renal artery stenosis and abdominal coarctation (Stringer *et al.*, 1984).

For all other situations Tc-DTPA is the radiopharmaceutical of choice.

Technique of Tc-DMSA scanning

Scanning times are shorter than for Tc-DTPA studies and infants will only rarely need sedation. Following intravenous injection of the agent (3.7 MBq kg^{-1}) approximately 50% of the administered dose is localized in the kidneys at 1 h and scanning is usually undertaken 2–6 h post injection. Renal activity reaches a plateau at 6 h and remains constant for 24 h so scanning at later times is possible.

A total of 300,000–500,000 counts is recorded in posterior and both posterior oblique projections. Anterior views are essential in the following situations:

1. When only one kidney is seen. With routine projections activity within a pelvic kidney is prevented from reaching the gamma camera because of absorption by the sacrum. This does not apply to the anterior projection (Figure 11.12).
2. When a horseshoe kidney is present, so that the spine does not obscure activity in the isthmus and lower poles.
3. Following renal transplantation. The transplanted kidney lies within the anterior abdomen.

Regions of interest are outlined for both kidneys and an area for background subtraction. Renal activity, after background subtraction, is counted and relative function calculated. In the presence of severe obstruction relative function may be overestimated due to the presence of some DMSA activity in the collecting system. Delayed images at 24 h will give a more accurate reflection of relative function because urinary activity will by that time have drained away but renal activity is still high.

Inflammatory disease

Acute pyelonephritis

$^{99m}Tc\text{-}DMSA$ Defects in renal activity which may be focal, multi-

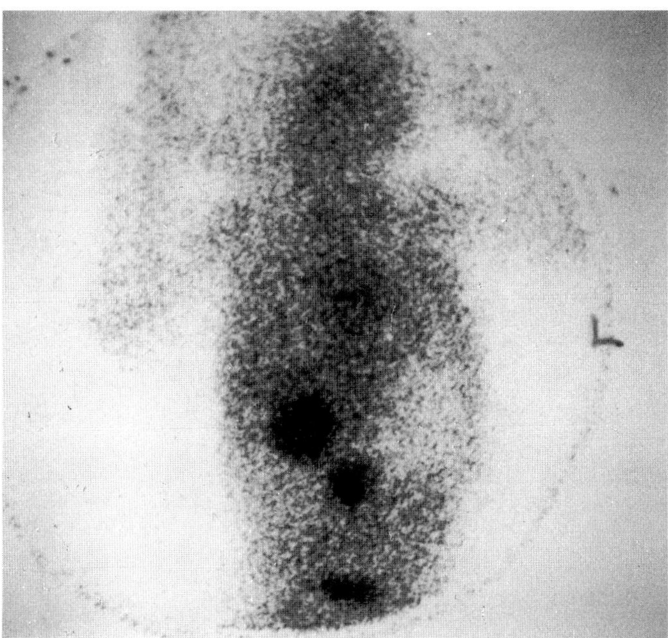

Figure 11.12 Tc-DMSA scan. Anterior view showing an ectopic left kidney in front of the spine. The large photon-deficient area in the left side of the abdomen is a full stomach

focal or generalized are seen in acute pyelonephritis and the scan is almost always abnormal in that condition. These defects in activity must not be confused with the normal foci of lower activity which correspond to the pelvicalyceal system. The EU has only a 25% sensitivity for acute pyelonephritis and an abnormal DMSA scan in the presence of a normal EU or ultrasound examination increases the probability of acute pyelonephritis (Handmaker, 1982). Early antibiotic treatment may allow the scan to return to normal but a persistent defect indicates the development of renal scarring. The DMSA scan will detect cortical loss before EU can show a change in cortical outline.

[67]Gallium citrate   Following an intravenous injection (80–160 MBq in adults) images are obtained at 24 h and 48 h when target-to-background ratios are optimal. After being cleared from the blood where it is bound to transferrin [67]gallium citrate localizes in polymorphs and in areas of high tissue concentration of lactofer-

rin, which is a major component of the soluble protein fraction of neutrophils. It has been shown to be 86% accurate in distinguishing upper from lower urinary tract infection (Hurwitz *et al.*, 1976). There are, however, a number of disadvantages:

1. Normal kidneys will take up gallium.
2. Activity within bowel may mask renal activity.
3. It is impossible to distinguish renal from extrarenal (i.e. perinephric) infections.
4. Acute tubular necrosis, vasculitis and leukaemic infiltration may also produce increased accumulation of gallium within the kidney.
5. The radiation dose is high.

^{111}Indium-labelled leucocytes   These are superior to ^{67}gallium citrate because any renal activity is indicative of infection and the radiation dose is lower. This method does have the disadvantage of the patient having to undergo a preliminary venepuncture to have autologous white cells removed.

Renal scarring
Tc-DMSA scanning has a greater sensitivity than urography for the

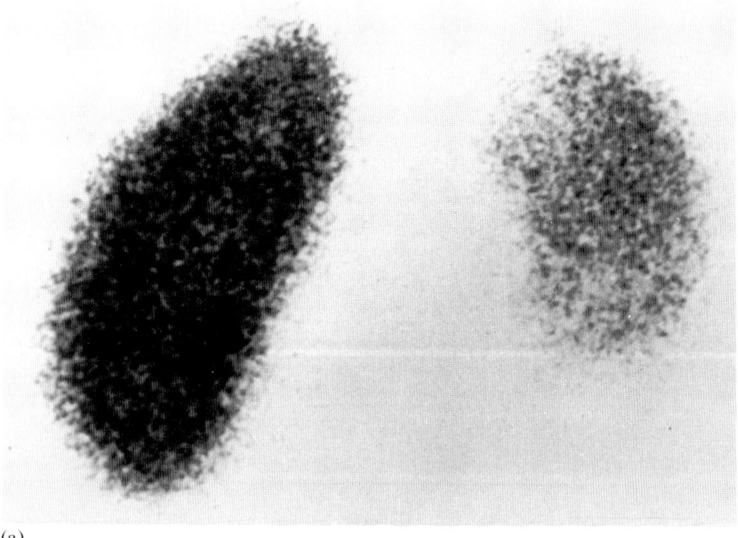

(a)

Figure 11.13 Tc-DMSA scan. Scarring shown on three projections. (a) Left posterior oblique. (b) Posterior. (c) Right posterior oblique views

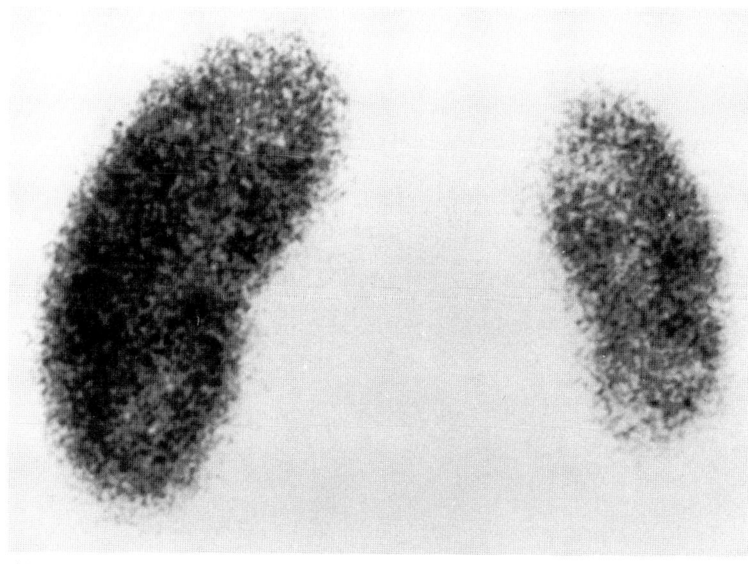

(b)

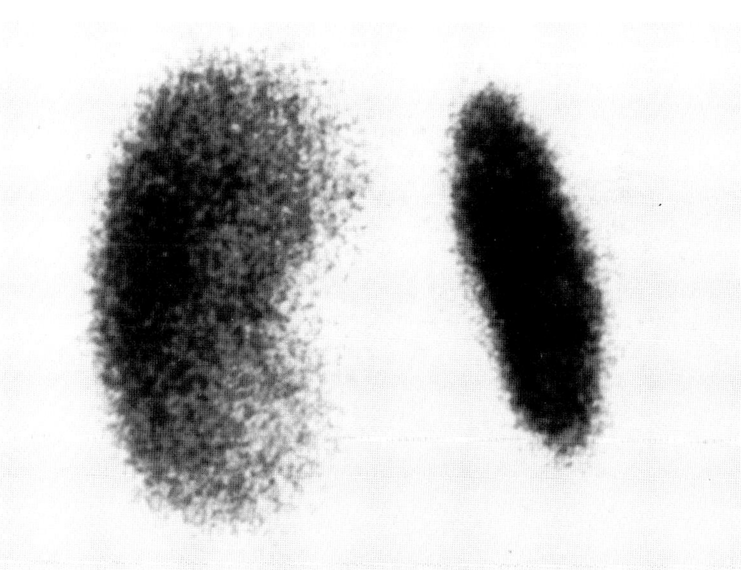

(c)

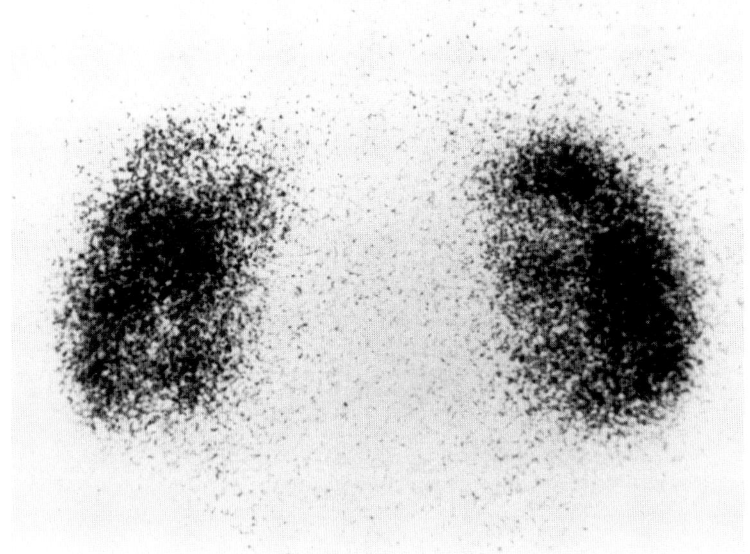

Figure 11.14 Tc-DMSA scan, single posterior view, showing multiple photon deficient areas due to bilateral renal scarring

detection of renal scarring. As in acute pyelonephritis the images show focal, multifocal or generalized defects in renal activity (Figures 11.13 and 11.14). Merrick, Utley and Wild (1980), in their study of renal scarring due to reflux nephropathy, found that EU had a sensitivity of 86% and a specificity of 92% while DMSA scanning had a sensitivity of 96% and a specificity of 98%. They concluded by saying that scan defects may precede radiological abnormalities and deterioration of follow-up radiographs may reveal only what is already visible on the earlier scans.

Reflux studies

The traditional method of choice for the detection of vesico-ureteric reflux is radiographic micturating cystourethrography (MCUG). It has the advantages of excellent delineation of anatomical abnormalities and accurate grading of reflux but is associated with a high gonadal radiation dose. In many paediatric centres radionuclide cystography (RNC) has replaced radiographic cystography for follow-up examinations.

Indications

1. Follow-up of known refluxers, including the postoperative evaluation of those who have had antireflux surgery.
2. Follow-up of children who are susceptible to the development of vesico-ureteric reflux, e.g. those with neuropathic bladders.
3. Screening of asymptomatic siblings of known refluxers.

There are two alternative methods.

Direct radionuclide cystography

This is technically similar to radiographic MCUG. The bladder is catheterized using aseptic technique and drained. The patient is positioned in front of the gamma camera with the field covering the bladder and renal areas. A small amount of sodium pertechnetate (20–40 MBq) is injected into the bladder followed by the instillation of sterile normal saline until micturition occurs. The examination is monitored on a persistence oscilloscope. Five-second frames are stored by the computer and analogue images are obtained during filling and micturition. If reflux is observed, regions of interest (ROI) are drawn around kidneys, bladder and a background area for subtraction. Time activity curves are generated for each ROI (Figure 11.15).

Advantages

1. Gonadal radiation dose during RNC may be reduced to one-hundredth that from X-ray cystography depending on the number of films taken during the latter investigation.
2. Greater sensitivity for the higher grades of reflux. Reflux is a dynamic but intermittent process and as RNC allows continuous monitoring of the urinary tract during the procedure, while radiation dosage during radiographic cystography limits the

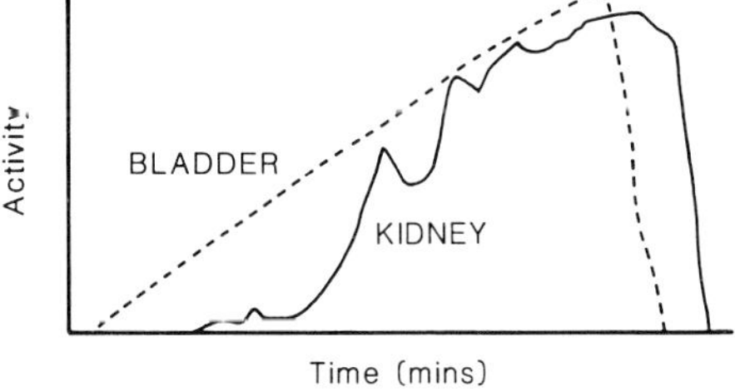

Figure 11.15 Direct radionuclide cystography. Time activity curve

observer to intermittent observation, the former should be more sensitive (Conway and Kruglik, 1976).

Disadvantages

1. The poor resolution of RNC compared with X-ray cystography means that anatomical abnormalities, e.g. urethral obstructions, ectopic ureters and ureterocoeles, cannot be evaluated. *Radionuclide cystography should not be used as the initial screening procedure for symptomatic children.*
2. Accurate grading of reflux is not possible and minor reflux into the lower end of the ureter will be obscured by radionuclide activity in the bladder.

Indirect radionuclide cystography

Direct radionuclide cystography requires bladder catheterization and may, therefore, be unpleasant for the patient. It also carries the small risk of introducing infection. To overcome these drawbacks an intravenous technique has been developed.

The procedure begins with a conventional Tc-DTPA renogram, thus providing additional information about renal function which retrograde cystography is incapable of demonstrating. The reflux part of the test does not begin until almost all the isotope has been excreted by the kidneys and the bladder is full of labelled urine. This occurs about 45–60 min after injection. The patient is repositioned, sitting in front of the gamma camera, and micturition allowed to occur into a commode or urine bottle. Sequential images are obtained from before the commencement of micturition until after it has ceased. Vesico-ureteric reflux is diagnosed when activity is seen in ureters or kidneys. Regions of interest are drawn around kidneys, bladder and a background area for subtraction and time activity curves generated for each ROI (Figure 11.16).

This technique has been shown to be more sensitive than radio-

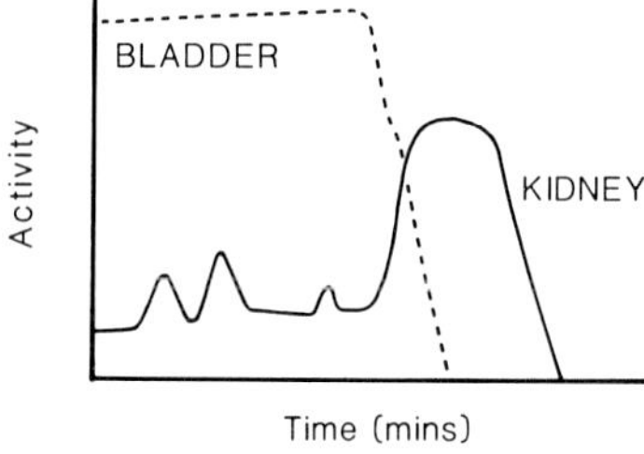

Figure 11.16 Indirect radionuclide cystography. Time–activity curve

graphic MCUG, and without the need for catheterization may be 'more physiological'. The main disadvantage is that it does require greater cooperation from the child, who needs to hold on to a full bladder and micturate on command. In addition impaired renal function and/or hydronephrosis can lead to retention of isotope in the kidneys, which may mask lesser degrees of reflux. Vesico-ureteric reflux may not be detected in the presence of high urine flow (Cremin, 1979) and thus to attempt indirect RNC after diuretic renography presents a conflict of methodology.

References and further reading

Radiopharmaceuticals
Treves, S. T., Lebowitz, R. L., Kuruc, A. *et al.* (1985) Kidneys. In *Pediatric Nuclear Medicine* (ed. S. T. Treves), Springer-Verlag, New York, pp. 63–103.

Dynamic imaging: renography
Jewkes, R. F. and Jayasingh, K. (1981) Comparison of ^{123}I-hippuran and ^{99m}Tc DTPA. *Nuclear Medicine Communications*, **2**, 278–288
O'Reilly, P. H. (1986) *Obstructive Uropathy*, Springer, Berlin, p. 73
O'Reilly, P. H., Shields, R. A. and Testa, H. J. (1987) *Nuclear Medicine in Urology and Nephrology*, 2nd edn, Butterworth, London
O'Reilly, P. H., Testa, H. J., Lawson, R. S. *et al.* (1978) Diuresis renography in equivocal urinary tract obstruction. *British Journal of Urology*, **50**, 76–80

Static renal imaging
Handmaker, H. (1982) Nuclear renal imaging in acute pyelonephritis. *Seminars in Nuclear Medicine*, **12**, 246–253
Hurwitz, S. R., Kessler, W. O., Alazraki, N. P. *et al.* (1976) Gallium-67 imaging to localise urinary-tract infections. *British Journal of Radiology*, **49**, 156–160
Merrick, M. V., Utley, M. S. and Wild, S. R. (1980) The detection of pyelonephritic scarring in children by radioisotope imaging. *British Journal of Radiology*, **53**, 544–546
Stringer, D. A., de Bruyn, R., Dillon, M. J. and Gordon, I. (1984) Comparison of aortography, renal vein sampling, radionuclide scans, ultrasound and the IVU in the investigation of childhood renovascular hypertension. *British Journal of Radiology*, **57**, 111–121

Reflux studies
Conway, J. J. (1984) Radionuclide cystography. In: Hodson, C. J., Heptinstall, J. and Winberg, J. (eds) *Contributions to Nephrology*, Vol. 39 (eds C. J. Hodson, J. Heptinstall and J. Winberg) Karger, Basel, pp. 1–19
Conway, J. J. and Kruglik, G. D. (1976) Effectiveness of direct and indirect radionuclide cystography in detecting vesicoureteral reflux. *Journal of Nuclear Medicine*, **17**, 81–83
Conway, J. J., Belman, A. B. and King, L. R. (1974) Direct and indirect radionuclide cystography. *Seminars in Nuclear Medicine*, **4**, 197–211
Cremin, B. J. (1979) Observations on vesico-ureteric reflux and intrarenal reflux. A review and survey of material. *Clinical Radiology*, **30**, 607–621

Chapter 12

Urodynamic investigations

Introduction

Urodynamic study is an extension of, not a substitute for, a careful micturition history and physical examination. Alone it does not determine whether a particular hydrodynamic abnormality is neuropathic or 'functional'; and this distinction, which is difficult in some children (Allen, 1977), has to be made on clinical grounds. One needs to remember that the bladder and urethra derive their innervation from sacral roots S3–S4. A micturition problem may be the first symptom of a corda equina lesion with no abnormal neurological sign in the legs. It is therefore important to test for perianal sensation, and assess tone and contractility of the pelvic floor. The perianal reflex, in which the anal margin is lightly stroked leading to involuntary contraction of the levator ani (the anal 'wink'), is a simple test of the integrity of the relevant sacral roots.

Patients with no apparent signs of neuropathy who present with daytime *urge incontinence*, perhaps following a urinary tract infection, seldom require dynamic investigation. These children, more often girls than boys, usually respond to simple management with frequent voiding and detrusor-relaxing drugs and there is a high rate of spontaneous improvement (de Jonge, 1973). Urodynamic evaluation should be reserved for those who fail to respond to treatment or who have evidence of an abnormal post-voiding residual urine volume – either a palpable/percussible bladder after voiding or a residual volume measured by ultrasound (Harrison, Parks and Sherwood, 1976).

All girls presenting with disturbances of daytime micturition should have a stress test as part of their physical examination. The child stands erect with a full bladder and is asked to bear down but resist voiding. Those in whom the manoeuvre causes incontinence (positive stress test) deserve dynamic study to confirm the diagnosis of *sphincter failure*. Radiographically these girls may be found to have the *wide bladder neck anomaly* (Stanton and Williams, 1973). The stress test by no means identifies all patients with this anomaly and others will come to light when urodynamic studies are applied to those small numbers of children with daytime incontinence who fail to respond to simple primary treatment. Careful inspection of the genitalia is essential in all incontinent children to identify urethral abnormalities and any signs of urine leakage from an aberrant site. An ultrasound scan of the upper urinary tract is a good screening test for a duplex system, which may point towards an ectopic ureter.

At present there is no place for urodynamic study in children with *nocturnal enuresis* only.

All children with *neuropathic bladders* should undergo evaluation as early as possible as the results point the way in which treatment may relieve urinary obstruction and promote continence. For example, urodynamic investigation is good at showing which children are likely to achieve continence and preserve upper tract morphology on a programme of clean intermittent bladder catheterization (Scott and Deegan, 1982), and it allows a rational approach to adjunctive medication or operative treatment (Borzyskowski and Mundy, 1988). Nowadays it is inappropriate to apply such treatments blindly.

Apparatus

Figure 12.1 shows the usual apparatus. Pressure is measured either by fluid-filled manometer lines connected to remote transducers or by microtransducers born on the tips of fine catheters. The pressure within the bladder has two components. The first is made up of the elastic and contractile property of the detrusor muscle itself, the second is the pressure transmitted to the bladder from the surrounding abdominal organs. Broadly speaking rectal pressure equates to the latter and so the rectal pressure is electronically subtracted from the intravesical pressure to reveal that component which is derived from detrusor itself. The three pressures are displayed separately on a multichannel recorder. To fill the bladder, saline is delivered via an accurate pump through a final urethral catheter. The volume instilled into the bladder is recorded either by a transducer attached to the bag of saline or, if the pump delivery rate is known, by time. For voiding studies there are various types of flow meter, all of which give a printout of flow rate against time on the recorder. The area under the curve is the voided volume and most machines calculate this at the end of the voiding study. The addition of simultaneous videocystourethrography is essential to the evaluation of some patients (Whiteside, 1972).

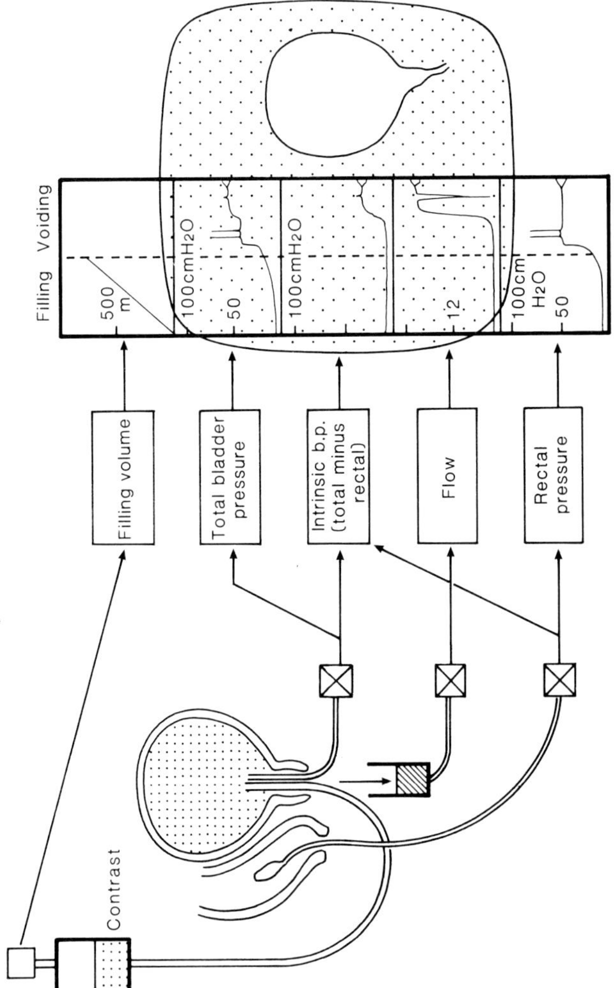

Figure 12.1 Schematic representation of urodynamic apparatus

Procedure

Apart from the measurement of urinary flow rates during voiding, urodynamic investigations involve catheterization and are therefore invasive procedures. Although elementary tests can be performed in infants and toddlers under sedation or light anaesthesia (Koff *et al.*, 1980), children are normally studied alert, which demands a high degree of trust and cooperation with the investigator. To achieve this children need to become familiarized with the diagnostic apparatus and its surroundings and to receive an appropriate explanation of the test. This psychological preparation is best performed by specially trained paediatric nursing staff and for these reasons urodynamic investigation should be confined to specialized paediatric centres. The following is therefore an outline of the technique for those who may need to refer patients rather than a blueprint for a developed service.

Urodynamic investigation must on no account become a painful procedure as a child who experiences urethral pain is likely to demonstrate artefactual voiding abnormalities. For this reason it is important not to study patients if they have recently had a symptomatic urinary infection. In boys undergoing voiding cystometry, and in any child with urethral hypersensitivity, bladder pressures should be measured by suprapubic catheter.

Combining dynamic measurements with cineradiography is useful, particularly in the study of patients with sphincter incompetence when surgical treatment is being considered. However, the radiation exposure to gonads is considerable and one can be selective over which patients have a combined study. Pelvic floor electromyography (EMG) using adhesive skin electrodes can give additional information in patients with bladder/sphincter dyssynergia (inappropriate urethral closure during voiding), and is popular in some centres. Needle electrode EMG is a further invasive escalation and should be reserved only for specific neurological tests. It has to be pointed out that each additional bit of apparatus applied to the child further divorces laboratory-observed micturition from that of ordinary life. In practice, the activity of the pelvic floor and the urethral sphincter can be judged well enough from the video recording in a combined radiographic study.

Free voiding studies
This simple non-invasive investigation can be repeated many times if necessary until a consistent pattern is seen. Children are asked to void into the uroflow meter when they sense the call to micturition. For girls a toilet seat is arranged over the meter. Boys normally

stand to void; those who elect to sit beyond the normal potty training stage are very likely to exhibit dyssynergia. In both sexes privacy is needed.

Children normally void in a continuous stream. Maximum urinary flow rates in any individual are dependent on the volume voided and are inversely proportional to the urethral resistance. Nomograms for normal ranges of maximal flow rate are available in adults but so far only one (Toguri, Uchida and Bee, 1982) has been provided for children. This suffers from the fact that it is standardized for body surface area and arbitrarily divided into children above and below $1.1m^2$, making it complicated to use. Using data from various sources Table 12.1 gives a broad guide to flow rate below which one would suspect a voiding disturbance.

The appearance of flow curve is often useful, different patterns being shown in Figure 12.2. Flow rates are used mostly as a screening test for outflow tract obstruction which may be a fixed anatomical lesion (posterior urethral valves, stricture, stenosis) or a functional obstruction associated with neuropathy or idiopathic 'bladder/sphincter dyssynergia'.

Residual urine

The residual urine volume can be calculated non-invasively using US (Harrison, Parks and Sherwood, 1976). If full urodynamic evaluation is to be performed, catheterization takes place immediately after voiding and the residual bladder urine is aspirated and measured. A consistently observed residual volume greater than 50 ml at any age, or more than 20% of bladder capacity, should be regarded as pathological.

Filling cystometry

This is a test of the reservoir function of the bladder. Normally the bladder is highly compliant so that on filling the detrusor pressure

Table 12.1   Least acceptable maximum urinary flow rate (ml s^{-1})

| | | Voided volume (ml) | | |
		100	150	> 200
Males	4–7 years	10	12	14
	8–12 years	12	15	17
	> 13 years	15	18	20
Females	4–7 years	11	13	15
	8–12 years	13	18	20
	> 13 years	15	20	22

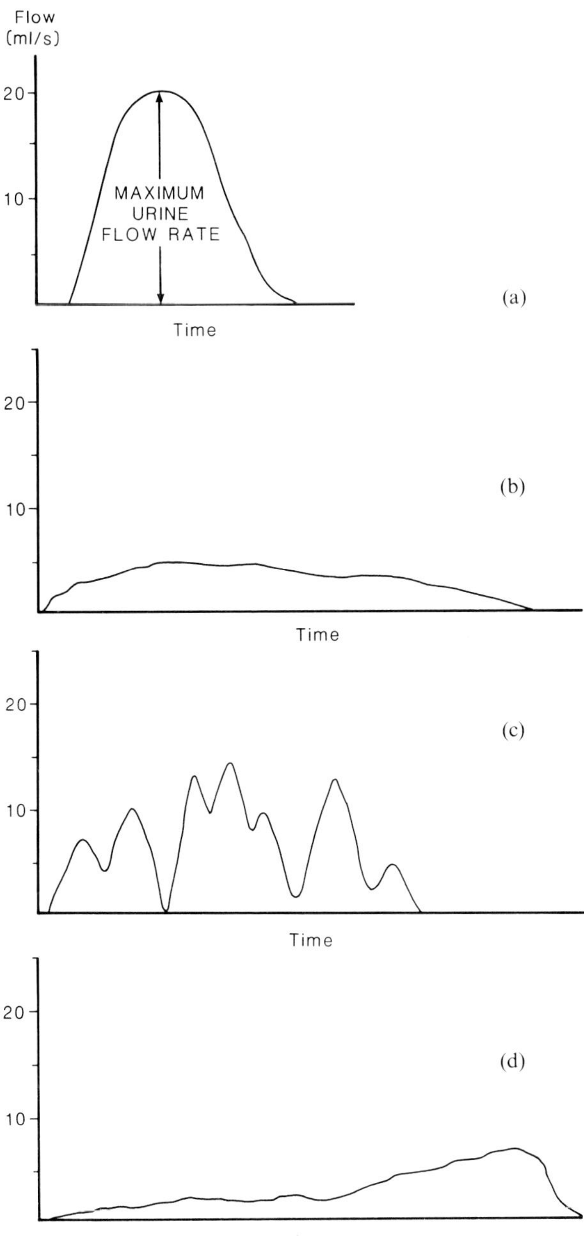

Figure 12.2 Urinary flow rates. (a) Normal. (b) Obstruction. (c) Bladder/sphincter dyssynergia. (d) Hypocontractility

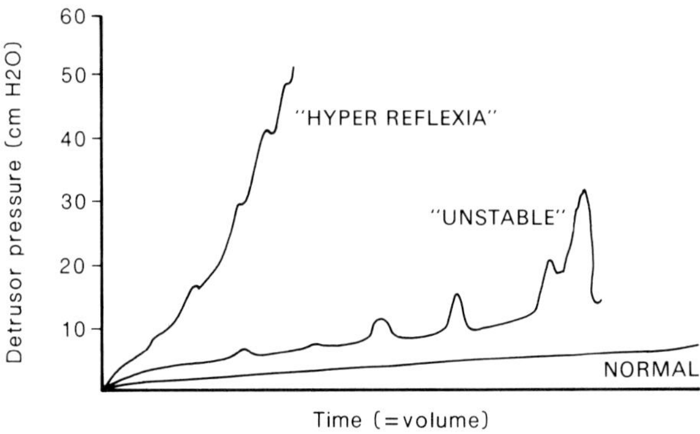

Figure 12.3 The cystometrogram

remains low, usually less than 10 cm of water pressure (Figure 12.3). The tidal capacity of the bladder, and the residual volume will be known from the child's previous voiding studies and catheterization respectively. During the cystometrogram (CMG) it is essential that the child cooperates with the instruction to 'hold on' and not void. This is impractical in children under 4 years of age in whom volition cannot be adjudicated.

The bladder is then filled with saline or contrast medium towards the anticipated capacity, during which the child communicates his or her bladder sensation to the investigator. The rate of filling for the initial CMG is usually 10 ml min^{-1} but this is not critical except for some neuropathic patients with detrusor hyperreflexia in whom the rate should be reduced. If the initial CMG shows compliance, it may be repeated with faster bladder filling and the patient erect. This manoeuvre is more likely to unmask detrusor contractions which this child is unable to suppress (unstable bladder).

The *filling* CMG gives information on bladder capacity and compliance. The normal bladder capacity in millilitres is approximately $(2 + \text{age in years}) \times 30$ (Koff, 1983). Functional capacity is often reduced because of uninhibitable bladder contractions (unstable bladder) and this is the typical dynamic finding in children with the urge incontinence syndrome. An unstable bladder does not by itself denote a neuropathy. Non-compliance may be neuropathic, as in the hyperreflexive bladder, myopathic or more rarely due to fibrosis and scarring.

Voiding cystometry
In children pressure/flow studies need careful interpretation. A good

guide is to compare the urinary flow rate and pattern with that observed during free voiding. Only if these are similar can reliance be placed on the pressure observations. During maximum urinary flow detrusor pressure is typically in the region of 40 ± 20 cm H_2O. A guide of the urethral resistance to flow may be calculated using the formula:

$$\text{Urethral resistance} = \sqrt{\frac{\text{voiding pressure at maximum flow}}{\text{maximum urine flow rate}}}.$$

The normal range for girls is < 0.58 cm H_2O ml^{-1} s^{-1} (Zatz, 1965). The range for boys is higher but poorly defined and depends on technique.

Fixed outflow tract obstruction is uncommon, except for posterior urethral valves in boys which are best diagnosed radiographically. Urodynamic investigation is better at picking up intermittent urinary tract obstruction during voiding – bladder/sphincter dyssynergia – in which the urethra may fail to relax or the pelvic diaphragm contracts inappropriately. This is seen in neuropathic patients but can also be an acquired functional problem. In the latter it is seen in those severely affected by the urge incontinence syndrome. These children habitually use their pelvic floor muscles to inhibit leakage. In addition to functional outflow tract obstruction, often with a urinary residuum, they develop constipation and recurrent urinary infection. The increased bladder work of voiding against a closed outlet gives rise to hypertrophy and high detrusor presssures during voiding which culminate in upper tract damage (Hinman, 1974).

Urethral closure pressure profile
For this test a special urethral catheter is used which has one or more side-holes arranged radially a few centimetres from its blind tip. The catheter is perfused with saline at a steady 2 ml min^{-1} and the pressure within is recorded with a transducer. The pressure of the urethra closing around the side-holes is reflected in the rise of pressure in perfusing fluid (Brown and Wickham, 1969).

The patient is catheterized in the supine position with the bladder empty. Once the side-holes are in the bladder the profile catheter is withdrawn at a steady slow speed with a tractor device and the contour of the closure pressure along the urethra is obtained (Figure 12.4). These contours are different between the sexes. In males one observes a prostatic plateau proximal to the main peak of closure pressure which occurs in the region of the membranous urethra. In girls the profile demonstrates the shorter urethra with a steep rise in pressure at the bladder neck and a symmetrical contour. In girls the

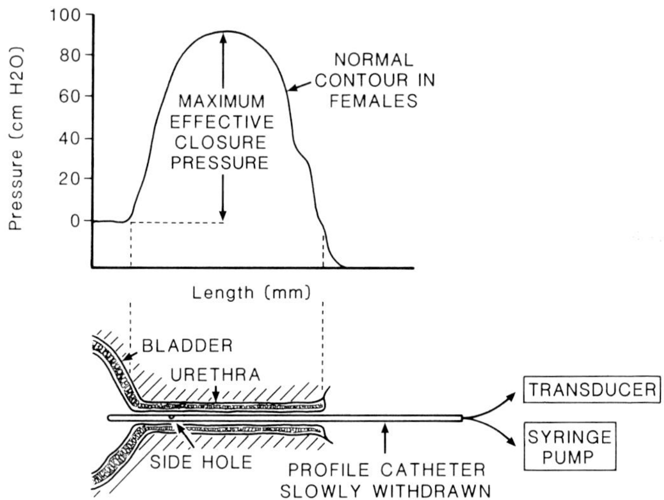

Figure 12.4 The urethral closure pressure profile

maximal effective closure pressure in mid-urethra is typically in the range of 60–100 cm · H_2O. In boys the range, although less well defined, appears to be wider; a maximal closure pressure below 50 cm H_2O is likely to be pathological.

About one-third of patients with neuropathic bladders show grossly defective urethral closure pressures. This test is also of use in evaluating girls with idiopathic stress incontinence, in whom the maximal pressure is often less than 45 cm H_2O with a shallow pressure rise in the proximal urethra.

Summary

- Flow rates are used to screen for outflow obstruction, especially detrusor/sphincter dyssynergia.
- Residual urine implies detrusor failure, obstruction or reflux.
- The CMG examines detrusor compliance during filling and contractility in voiding.
- The voiding CMG identifies dyssynergia.
- The urethral closure pressure profile is useful in stress incontinence.
- Every child with clinical evidence of a neuropathic bladder deserves early dynamic investigation so that treatment can be offered to prevent renal damage and to promote continence.

References

Allen, T. D. (1977) The non-neurogenic neurogenic bladder. *Journal of Urology*, **117**, 232–238

Borzyskowski, M. and Mundy, A. R. (1988) The management of the neuropathic bladder in childhood. *Pediatric Nephrology*, **2**, 56–66

Brown, M. and Wickham, J. E. A. (1969) The urethral pressure profile. *British Journal of Urology*, **41**, 211–217

de Jonge, G. A. (1973) The urge syndrome. In *Bladder Control and Enuresis* (eds I. Kolvin, R. C. MacKeith and S. R. Meadow), *Clinics in Developmental Medicine*, 48/49, Heinemann, London, pp. 66–69

Harrison, N. W., Parks, C. and Sherwood, T. (1976) Ultrasound assessment of residual urine in children. *British Journal of Urology*, **47**, 805–814

Hinman, F. (1974) Urinary tract damage in children who wet. *Pediatrics*, **54**, 142–150

Koff, S. A. (1983) Estimating bladder capacity in children. *Urology*, **21**, 245

Koff, S. A., Solomon, M. H., Lane, G. A. *et al.* (1980) Urodynamic studies in anaesthetised children. *Journal of Urology*, **123**, 61–63

Scott, J. E. S. and Deegan, S. (1982) Management of neuropathic urinary incontinence in children by intermittent catheterisation. *Archives of Disease in Childhood*, **57**, 253–258

Stanton, L. and Williams, D. I. (1973) The wide bladder neck in children. *British Journal of Urology*, **45**, 60–64

Toguri, A. G., Uchida, T. and Bee, D. E. (1982) Pediatric uroflowrate nomograms. *Journal of Urology*, **127**, 727–731

Whiteside, C. G. (1972) Videocystographic studies with simultaneous pressure and flow recordings. *British Medical Bulletin*, **28**, 214–219

Zatz, I. M. (1965) Combined physiologic and radiological studies of bladder function in female children with recurrent urinary tract infections. *Investigative Urology*, **3**, 278–308

Further reading

Abrams, P., Fenely, R. and Torrens, M. (1983) *Urodynamics*, Springer-Verlag, Berlin, Heidelberg, New York.

Chapter 13

Renal biopsy

Percutaneous renal biopsy has become a safe and reliable procedure in paediatric nephrology, and now the only place for open biopsy is during coincidental renal surgery. Its safety stems from the fact that haemostasis and urine sterility are checked beforehand and that the kidney is visualized during sampling either by excretion urography or ultrasound. These precautions minimize the chance of traumatizing the vascular pedicle of the kidney, perforating a calyx or running into problems with haemorrhage. With the advent of real-time ultrasound a 'blind' renal biopsy is no longer acceptable practice. The procedure is usually done under local anaesthesia and children therefore require confident nursing and sedation; we have found promazine and pethidine 1 mg kg^{-1} to be satisfactory. General anaesthesia is only needed for vigorous toddlers.

The disposable Tru-Cut (Travenol Laboratories) biopsy needle is the easiest to use and causes minimal distortion of the sample core (White and Jivani, 1974). The tissue obtained is inspected with a dissecting microscope immediately after collection to discern areas of cortex and medulla. With the trained eye one can identify glomeruli in the former, whereas the medulla has a streaky appearance because of the parallel vasa recta. The core can then be divided for light microscopy, immunofluorescence and electron microscopy ensuring that glomeruli are present in each piece. The renal biopsy technique can be mastered readily, but as with other invasive procedures one needs to practise it regularly to maintain a high operative standard, and for these reasons it should only be performed in centres recognized for their paediatric nephrological expertise. Moreover there needs to be close liaison between clinician and pathologist so that the histological appearances are interpreted appropriately. Taken in isolation the biopsy may not allow a disease process to be classified satisfactorily, and it is only when other clinical and laboratory evidence is taken into account that a working diagnosis can be reached. For example, the histological finding of focal segmental glomerulosclerosis could relate to either an idiopathic nephrotic syndrome or 'remnant kidney' and renal insufficiency resulting from a wide range of destructive processes.

This chapter outlines some of the indications for biopsy and gives an overview of possible diagnostic end-points. The accompanying glossary (Table 13.1) and illustrations (Figures 13.1–13.4) provide a simple guide to commonly used histological terms.

Table 13.1   Glossary of histological terms

Minimal change	Normal appearance by light microscopy. By electron microscopy, fusion of foot processes, a non-specific and reversible response to proteinuria.
Proliferation	Increase in cell numbers, cell type to be defined. Example mesangial proliferation; > 3 cells per mesangial area.
Exudation	Infiltrated by neutrophils. Example acute post-streptococcal nephritis.
Membranous	Refers to the capillary wall or more specifically the glomerular basement membrane.
Hyalinosis	Insudation and condensation of plasma proteins into tissues outside a blood vessel lumen.
Sclerosis	Structureless material obliterating collapsed capillaries; equivalent to scar tissue.
Tubular atrophy	Thickening and wrinkling of tubular basement membrane; implies tubular ischaemia and loss of the nephron.
Crescent	In the early stages proliferation of epithelial cells of Bowman's capsule later replaced by fibrin, encompassing the glomerular tuft.
Diffuse	Applying to all glomeruli or all parts of a glomerulus in a biopsy.
Focal	Applying to some glomeruli not others.
Global	Applying to the whole of a glomerulus.
Segmental	Applying to part of a glomerulus, i.e. some capillaries unaffected.
'Humps'	Deposits of Ig and complement in a subepithelial site; typical of acute post-streptococcal nephritis.
'Spikes'	Projections of basement membrane between deposits, typical of membranous nephropathy.
Foam cells	Lipid laden cells, histiocytes, mesangial or tubular cells, seen in nephrotic syndrome and Alport's syndrome.

Stains for light microscopy

Haematoxylin and eosin (H and E). This stains cytoplasm pink and nuclei blue. It is often used to inspect for interstitial infiltration. It allows inspection of all renal structures but is poor at distinguishing deposits or showing changes in basement membrane. PAS counterstained with haematoxylin is often preferred.

Silver/periodic acid Schiff (PAS). PAS is a useful counterstain to silver staining and shows all cytoplasm in puce. The silver stain fixes to reticulin, basement membrane, collagen and fibrous material and appears black.

Martius scarlet blue (MSB). This is a useful stain which shows up proteinaceous insudative lesions, deposits or fibrin in red and collagen in blue. Erythrocytes appear yellow.

Toluidine blue. This stain is often used to screen tissues prior to preparing them for electron microscopy.

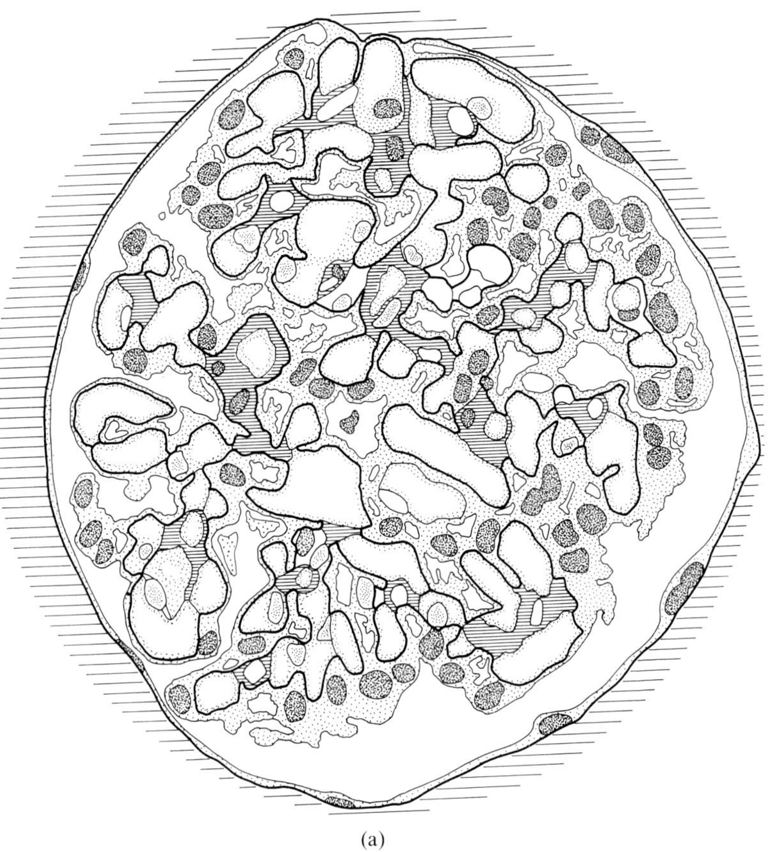

(a)

Figure 13.1 (a) Normal glomerulus by light microscopy. The hilum is at 12 o'clock. The hatched areas show mesangium, light stippling the epithelial and endothelial cell cytoplasm and dark stippling the nuclei. Note that in any mesangial area there are less than three mesangial nuclei.

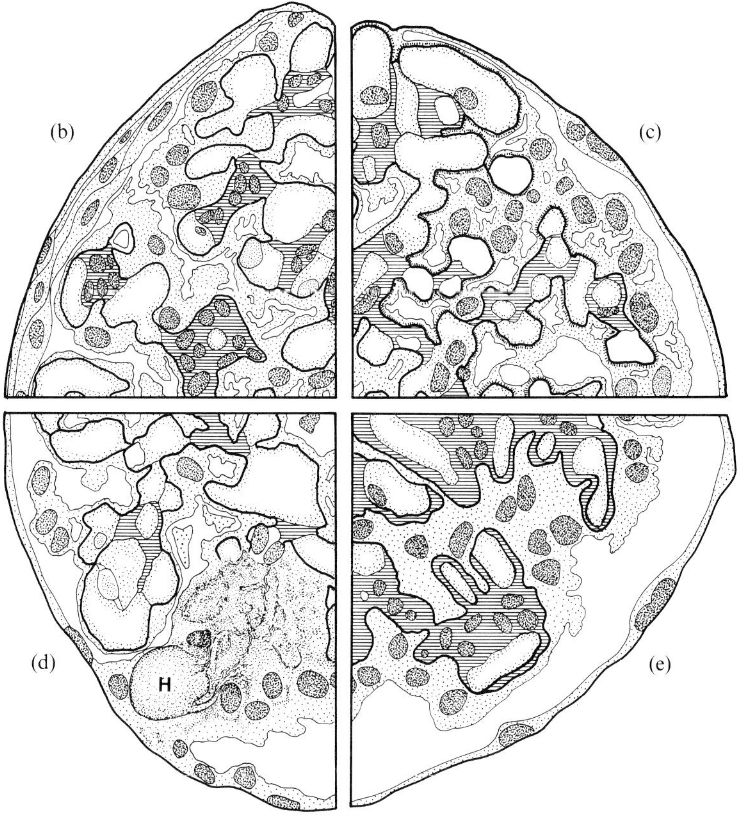

Figure 13.1 (*cont.*) (b) This shows proliferation of mesangial cells, and the epithelial cells of Bowman's capsule are replicating to form a crescent. As a diffuse lesion this may be seen in Henoch–Schönlein purpura, IgA nephropathy, post-infectious glomerulonephritis and in some forms of infantile onset nephrotic syndrome. (c) Membranous nephropathy. In this early lesion the spikes of basement membrane-like material are seen to project on the epithelial side of the capillary. This is best seen with a silver stain. At this stage no destructive lesion in the glomerulus is shown. (d) Focal glomerulosclerosis. Here an adhesion has formed between the sclerotic lesion and Bowman's capsule. In the sclerotic area capillary loops have collapsed completely and there is loss of nuclei. A droplet of hyaline (H) is seen. (e) Membranoproliferative glomerulonephritis. In this lesion there is proliferation of mesangial cells and matrix. The mesangium spreads out underneath the endothelial cells and a new layer of basement membrane is formed giving rise to the double contour of the capillaries. This is best seen with a silver stain. The capillary lumens become compressed and the capillary tuft appears dense.

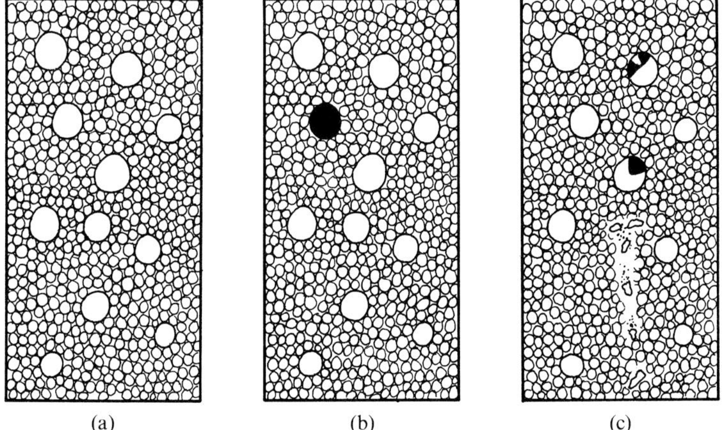

(a)   (b)   (c)

Figure 13.2 At low power (a) normal glomeruli and tubules are seen throughout the section. In (b) a glomerulus is totally sclerosed or obsolescent while neighbouring glomeruli are unaffected. This contrasts with (c) where there are focal segmental lesions and an area of tubular atrophy.

Nephrotic syndrome

Over 85% of children with the nephrotic syndrome have *minimal change disease*. They usually first present between the ages of 1 and 6 years and are most readily identified by the absence of hypertension and haematuria, and normal renal function. Treatment with prednisolone 2 mg kg^{-1} day^{-1} typically induces a remission within 4 weeks (an abrupt loss of proteinuria on early morning urine Albustix testing). There is no need to biopsy these steriod-responsive patients. There is a small population of children with minimal change nephrotic syndrome who respond to steroids between 4 and 8 weeks, so-called late responders, and rarely children with this histological diagnosis fail to respond at all (steroid-resistant nephrotic syndrome). However, the longer a patient is treated with prednisolone beyond 4 weeks without remission, the greater the likelihood of an alternative diagnosis such as focal segmental glomerulosclerosis. Focal segmental sclerosis is the second commonest diagnostic group accounting for up to 7% in some unselected series (White, Glasgow and Mills, 1970; International Study of Kidney Disease in Children, 1978). It seems to be a reasonable policy, therefore, to offer a biopsy to any child with a primary nephrotic syndrome who has failed to enter remission after 4 weeks of steriods, and by 8 weeks it is mandatory.

The onset of nephrotic syndrome before 1 year of age is uncommon, and within that group are those with *congenital or familial* disorders. Nephrological referral is indicated and a renal biopsy is helpful in distinguishing some of the underlying diseases. For example, the Finnish type of congenital nephrotic syndrome bears the hallmark of microcystic changes in the tubules of the deeper cortex (Huttunen, 1976), and is unlike other histological forms such as diffuse mesangial sclerosis (Habib and Bois, 1973) or focal segmental glomerular sclerosis.

Nephrotic patients with persistent hypocomplementaemia, usually older children and adults, are likely to have *membrano-proliferative glomerulonephritis*. This disease, which appears to be getting rarer, is readily diagnosed histologically and can be subdivided into two main types (White, 1978; see Figures 13.3 and 13.4). *Membranous nephropathy* is rare in childhood in North America and Western Europe. It appears to be more prevalent in South-east Asia where it is associated with hepatitis B antigenaemia. Approximately half of these patients present with heavy proteinuria and their failure to respond promptly to steroid becomes the indication for biopsy.

Vasculopathy

The haemolytic uraemic syndromes
This heterogeneous disorder is now the commonest cause of acute renal failure in children in North America and Western Europe (Fong, de Chadarevian and Kaplan, 1982). In 95% of patients it develops as a complication of an enteric infection, of which the leading cause is verotoxin-producing *E. coli* (Karmali *et al.*, 1985). In these post-enteropathic patients there is little value in performing histology as it can only be performed safely once the thrombocytopenia has resolved and it provides no additional guidance to the acute management. The prognosis can in part be anticipated histologically in that patients with involvement of large arteries or extensive cortical necrosis are more likely to have a poor outcome than those with just glomerular endothelial lesions.

Children who have *non-prodromal* haemolytic uraemic syndrome and those with a family history have a much more serious disease, 80% of them progressing to end-stage renal failure or death. Some respond to plasmapheresis, and in these histology is useful in monitoring the clinical course.

Henoch–Schönlein purpura and nephritis
Almost all patients with Henoch–Schönlein purpura have microscopic haematuria at some time during the course of their illness and

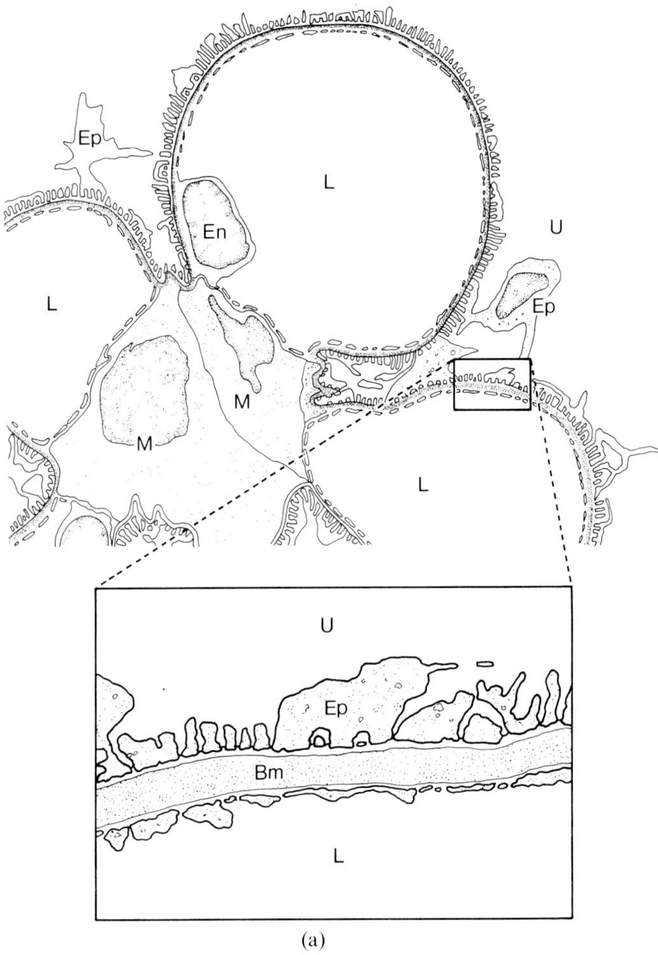

Figure 13.3 (a) A normal ultrastructural appearance at low and high power.
Ep = epithelial cell, En = endothelial cell, M = mesangial cell, L = lumen of capillary,
U = urinary space, Bm = basement membrane.

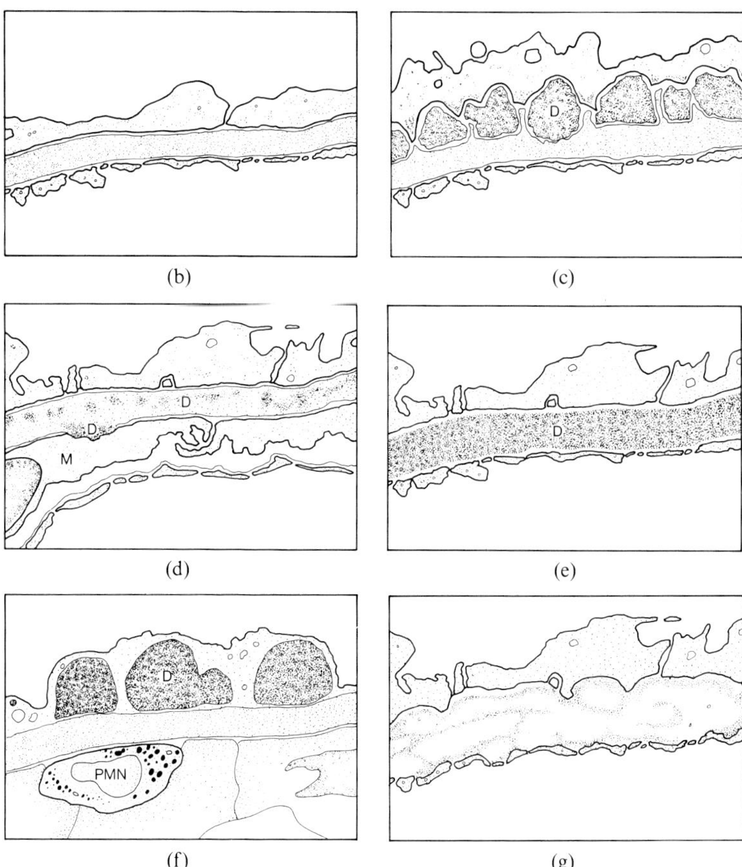

Figure 13.3 (b) Foot process fusion has occurred as a reaction to heavy protein-uria. This may be the only abnormality to be found in minimal change nephrotic syndrome. (c) Membranous nephropathy. The basement membrane is expanded by deposit (D) and there are little extensions of the normal basement membrane lamina densa between deposits and it is these which appear as spikes on light microscopy. (d) Membranoproliferative glomerulonephritis. Here there is extensive deposition of immune material throughout the basement membrane and there is mesangial cell (M) interposition between the basement membrane and the under-lying endothelium. (e) Dense deposit disease (also known as membranoproliferative glomerulonephritis Type II). Here the lamina densa is replaced and expanded by dense deposit. (f) Acute post-streptococcal glomerulonephritis. Humps of immune deposit are seen on the epithelial surface of the basement membrane. In the acute phase there is proliferation of many cells and leucocyte infiltration. A polymorphonuclear cell (PMN) is seen between the basement membrane and the endothelium. (g) Alport's syndrome. This shows the characteristic basement membrane abnormality. There are extensive lucent areas and the lamina densa is replicated giving rise to a 'basket weave' pattern. The epithelial surface of the basement membrane is bosselated and the membrane is thicker than normal.

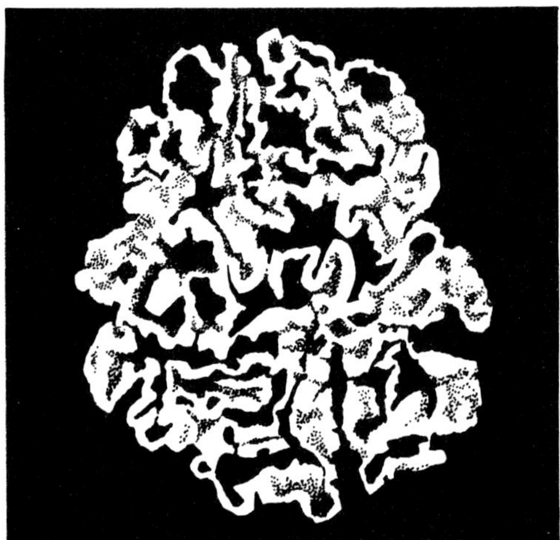

Figure 13.4 Immunofluorescence. Here a glomerulus stained for IgG shows diffuse granular deposition throughout the capillary walls. Such a finding is seen in membranous or membranoproliferative glomerulonephritis. In some forms of membranous nephropathy the appearance is less granular and more ribbon-like. A similar appearance when staining for IgA can be seen in Henoch–Schönlein purpura, but usually with more clumps of fluorescence and in IgA nephropathy the lesion is more often mesangial.

thus evidence of renal involvement. Those who, at the end of the acute phase, have only microscopic haematuria and no proteinuria can be expected to make a full recovery. The heavier the proteinuria on follow-up, the greater the likelihood of a progressive glomerular lesion (Counahan *et al.*, 1977). Biopsy is therefore indicated in patients who have impaired GFR or who are nephrotic at onset, and those with heavy proteinuria (early morning urine (EMU) protein/ creatinine ratio > 200 mg mmol^{-1}) at 8 weeks of follow-up.

The typical histological findings are those of a focal proliferative nephritis with IgA and complement C_3 deposited in the mesangium or capillary walls. With increasing severity a diffuse proliferative lesion and crescent formation are seen. The percentage of glomeruli affected by crescents gives a useful prognosis, more than 75% indicating a grave outlook.

Systemic lupus erythematosus
Approximately 80% of children with systemic lupus erythematosus have some form of renal involvement and it is predominantly this that determines the child's outcome. A wide range of histological

appearances may be seen ranging from mild mesangial proliferation, sometimes focal in distribution, through membranous lupus nephritis to a diffuse proliferative lesion with marked endothelial and mesangial hypercellularity and leucocyte infiltration. It is in the latter group that the renal prognosis is particularly poor. In that a fine balance has to be maintained between the benefits and risks of long-term immunosuppressive treatment and the variable disease activity, the biopsy findings give useful guidance (Rush *et al.*, 1986).

Nephritis

Although the prevalence of *acute post-streptococcal glomeruloneph-ritis* has declined, it remains a common illness. The disease is often subclinical but in those children who come to medical notice the typical clinical features are facial oedema, haematuria, pallor and hypertension. The prognosis is usually good and renal biopsy is reserved for those patients with an atypical presentation or clinical course. It is an urgent matter to identify those rare patients with a crescentic nephritis who rapidly progress to chronic renal failure. If during the acute presentation a child has anuria or a profound reduction in GFR, or a superimposed nephrotic syndrome an urgent biopsy is indicated. In typical post-streptococcal glomerulonephritis there is a prompt resolution of the illness and therefore patients whose renal impairment or hypertension persists beyond 2–3 weeks need a definitive diagnosis. Also, if the depression of complement C_3 persists beyond 6 weeks it suggests an alternative diagnosis such as membranoproliferative glomerulonephritis and again a biopsy is needed (Travis, 1978).

In the invesigation of a child with isolated *persistent microscopic haematuria*, which points to a chronic glomerulonephritis, one needs to consider familial disorders such as Alport's syndrome as well as acquired lesions. In the former it is imperative to screen family members with Haemastix, and in male subjects perform an audiogram. Alport's syndrome is usually an X-linked recessive so that boys express the full disease; mothers may be symptomless but have microscopic haematuria. Our recent experience has been that carriers may have intermittent haematuria only and therefore screening needs to be repeated. Electron microscopy is essential for revealing the characteristic replication of the lamina densa of the capillary basement membrane.

Acquired persistent haematuria is most likely to be due to IgA nephropathy, for which immunofluorescent staining techniques are needed, or the early presentation of focal segmental glomeruloneph-ritis. Some patients have minor and poorly defined abnormalities and a clear histological diagnosis cannot be made. It is common practice not to biopsy children with isolated *intermittent* haematuria as the diagnostic yield is smaller and the prospect of finding a progressive disease is remote. The finding of significant proteinuria, however, is a different matter and raises the probability of a destructive glomerular lesion, therefore patients should be monitored by infrequent quantification of proteinuria (see Chapter 4).

Miscellaneous

Histology can be valuable in interstitial nephritis, cystic renal disease and infiltrated disorders such as amyloidosis. It is also valuable in diabetic patients with proteinuria to distinguish diabetic nephropathy from other coexisting renal disease.

Summary

- In a nephrotic patient haematuria, hypertension, raised jugular venous pressure and impaired GFR are not typical of minimal change disease and their appearance is an indication for biopsy.
- In a nephritic illness the heavier the proteinuria the more extensive the glomerular lesion, raising the need for early histological guidance.

References

Counahan, R. Winterborn, M. H., Meadow, S. R. *et al.* (1977) The prognosis of Schönlein–Henoch nephritis. *British Medical Journal*, **2**, 11–14

Fong, J. S. C., de Chadarevian, J.-P. and Kaplan, B. S. (1982) Hemolytic-uremic syndrome. Current concepts and management. *Pediatric Clinics of North America*, **29**, 835–856.

Habib, R. and Bois, E. (1973) Hétérogénéité des syndromes nephrotiques a début précoce du nourrisson (syndrome nephrotique 'infantile'). *Helvetica Paediatrica Acta*, **28**, 91–107

Huttunen, N. P. (1976) Congenital nephrotic syndrome of the Finnish type: study of 75 patients. *Archives of Disease in Childhood*, **51**, 344–348

International Study of Kidney Disease in Children (1978) The nephrotic syndrome in children. Prediction of histopathology from clinical and laboratory characteristics at the time of diagnosis. *Kidney International*, **13**, 159–165

Karmali, M. A., Petric, M., Lim, C. *et al.* (1985) The association between idiopathic hemolytic uremic syndrome and infection by verotoxin-producing *Escherichia coli*. *Journal of Infectious Disease*, **151**, 775–782

Rush, P. J., Baumal, R., Shore, A. *et al.* (1986) Correlation of renal histology with outcome in children with lupus nephritis. *Kidney International*, **29**, 1066–1071

Travis, L. B. (1978) Acute postinfectious glomerulonephritis. In *Pediatric Kidney Disease* (ed. C. M. Edelmann), Little, Brown and Company, Boston, pp. 611–631

White, R. H. R. (1978) Membranoproliferative glomerulonephritis. In *Pediatric Kidney Disease* (ed. C. M. Edelmann), Little, Brown and Company, Boston, pp. 660–679

White, R. H. R. and Jivani, S. K. M. (1974) Evaluation of a disposable needle for renal biopsy in children. *Clinical Nephrology*, **2**, 120–122

White, R. H. R., Glasgow, E. F. and Mills, R. J. (1970) Clinicopathological study of nephrotic syndrome in childhood. *Lancet*, i, 1353–1359.

Problem-related investigation schemes

Urinary tract infection

Whereas the onset of dysuria, incontinence, urgency and frequency of micturition are strong indicators of urinary tract infection (UTI) in children of school age, such symptoms cannot be used in the very young. Infants with urinary infection are more likely to exhibit irritability and feeding problems, and neonates may present with jaundice. Astute mothers may notice that a baby's urinary stream is abnormal, a stop/start flow or small dribbles of urine rather than a complete void. Patients with a fever of more than 38.5°C or an elevated plasma concentration of C-reactive protein are much more likely to have renal parenchymal involvement (acute pyelonephritis) than uncomplicated lower urinary tract infection (Jodal, Lindberg and Lincoln, 1975). However, the absence of pyrexia does not exclude renal parenchymal disease in infancy.

It is well recognized that below 3 years of age children with infection are much more likely to develop renal scarring (Berg and Johansson, 1983). Although there may be age-dependent biological reasons for this, it seems likely that difficulty in making the diagnosis in children who are not yet toilet trained and delay in starting treatment are major factors. Animal experiments show that there is only a short period in which to clear bacteria from the renal interstitium before the inflammatory lesion inevitably heals by fibrosis (Ransley and Risdon, 1981).

In Figure A1.1 patients are divided, therefore, according to age and symptomatology. In infants, preschool children or any patient with fever or loin pain, urgent microscopy of freshly collected urine is mandatory. The presence of bacteria or excess leucocytes may be taken as an indication to start treatment without waiting for culture confirmation. By contrast, in older patients with only the signs and symptoms of lower urinary tract infection it is reasonable to await culture results before accepting the diagnosis and starting treatment. If, in the latter group of patients, microscopy in primary care practice is not immediately available a positive nitrite test on a freshly collected urine sample, together with a dip slide culture, will support the diagnosis.

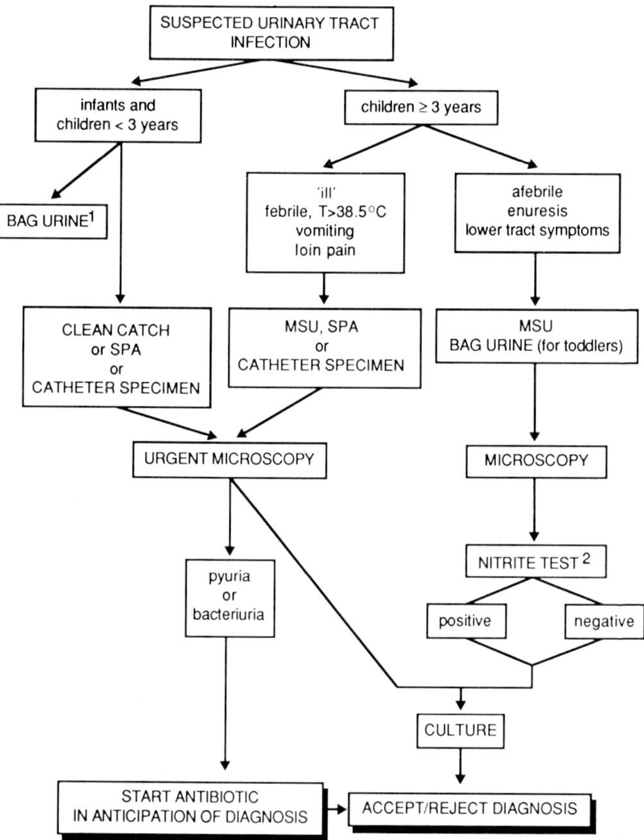

Figure A1.1 Algorithm for the investigation of suspected urinary tract infection.
[1]A bag urine sample which on microscopy contains no organisms or leucocytes makes UTI unlikely but does not exclude it. [2]A similar culture result is required from two consecutive MSU/bag urine samples for a confident diagnosis of UTI. However, a positive nitrite test sufficiently increases the probability of the diagnosis that a single culture result may be accepted

For children of any age successful diagnosis and treatment depend absolutely on the appropriate method of urine collection as discussed in Chapter 1.

All children who have had an episode of proven urinary tract infection deserve imaging, and the non-invasive nature of ultrasonography (US) makes this the ideal first investigation. Unlike excretion urography (EU), interpretation is more observer dependent. Nevertheless a formal comparison has shown that obstruction and major renal abnormalities can be identified with confidence, and it is

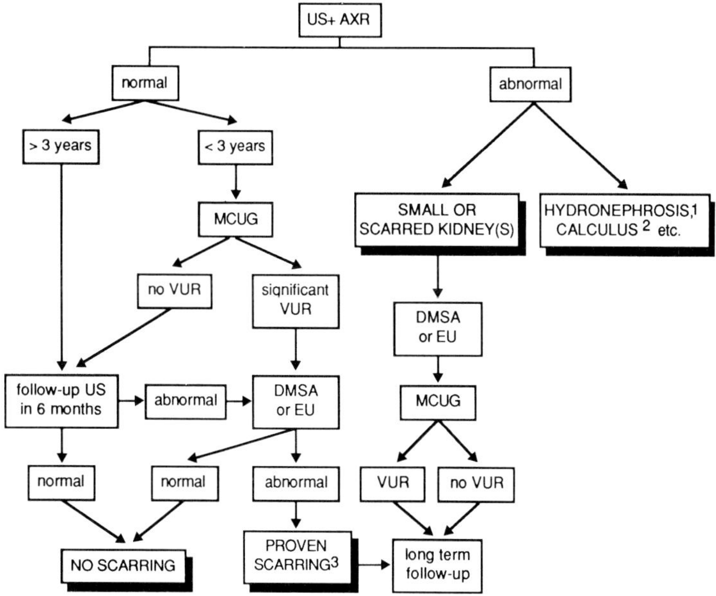

Figure A1.2 Algorithm for imaging following urinary tract infection. [1]See management of the dilated renal pelvis in Appendix 6. [2]See Appendix 5. [3]MCUG is indicated if not already performed

only with small scars or minor calyceal blunting that precision is reduced (Lindsell and Moncrieff, 1986). The addition of a plain abdominal X-ray increases the possibility of finding urinary calculi and allows spinal abnormalities to be seen.

The fibrous contraction of scarring may take several months to develop so that imaging close to the time of renal parenchymal infection may miss a new scar. We therefore recommend a follow-up ultrasound scan for all normal kidneys at 6 months.

Because the risk of scarring is strongly associated with both vesico-ureteric reflux (VUR) and the first 3 years of life, it is within this age-group that we recommend children should undergo micturating cystourethrography (MCUG). Probably the simplest scoring system for grades of severity of VUR is that devised by Rolleston, Shannon and Utley (1970). In grade I contrast medium is seen in the lower ureter, in grade II it reaches the pelvicalyceal system but without dilatation, and in grade III the calyces are distended when compared with the excretion urogram. In practice it is only grade III, and rarely grade II VUR which is associated with further *new* scar formation and therefore regarded as 'significant'.

Having identified severe reflux, or if US suggests the presence of scarring, further imaging is useful to define the renal morphology more accurately. The choice between EU and DMSA scan depends largely on local experience with each technique. Excretion urography gives detail of the calyces and ureters, the latter being useful if surgery is considered. Close to the time of the urinary infection a DMSA scan has the advantage of disclosing cold areas before scar contraction takes place, and thus anticipates later urographic changes.

Patients with severe reflux should be identified and treated as early in life as possible. Two forms of management are commonly used: ureteric reimplantation or low-dose antibiotic chemoprophylaxis until reflux resolves or the child outgrows the risk period. There is no overwhelming advantage of one form of treatment over the other (Birmingham Reflux Study Group, 1987). Following appropriate treatment, the aim is to decide which of the following three final outcome groups pertain to the patient (White and Taylor, 1984).

No renal scarring
So long as the child has outgrown the risk period for developing new scars, the prognosis for normal function is excellent and the chance of developing hypertension is that of the normal population. Such children can be discharged from medical supervision.

Unilateral scarring with a normal contralateral kidney
These patients have normal renal function at least in childhood and early adult life because of compensatory function by the unaffected kidney. They do, however, have approximately a 1 in 8 chance of developing hypertension over 20 years of follow-up; therefore, they need blood pressure monitoring within the setting of primary care.

Bilateral scarring
Where there is extensive loss of renal tissue renal function may be reduced and show a progressive decline. The hypertension risk is also higher. Such patients need to be monitored in a nephrological clinic.

References and further reading

Berg, U. B. and Johansson, S.B. (1983) Age as a determinant of renal functional damage in urinary tract infection. *Archives of Disease in Childhood*, **58**, 963–969
Birmingham Reflux Study Group (1987) Prospective trial of operative versus non-operative treatment of severe vesicoureteric reflux in children: five years' observation. *British Medical Journal*, **295**, 237–241

Haycock, G. B. (1986) Investigation of urinary tract infection. *Archives of Disease in Childhood*, **61**, 1155–1158

Jodal, U., Lindberg, U. and Lincoln, K. (1975) Level diagnosis of symptomatic urinary tract infection in childhood. *Acta Paediatrica Scandinavica*, **64**, 201–208

Lindsell, D. and Moncrieff, M. (1986) Comparison of ultrasound examination and intravenous urography after a urinary tract infection. *Archives of Disease in Childhood*, **61**, 81–82

Ransley, P. G. and Risdon, R. A. (1981) Reflux nephropathy: effects of antimicrobial therapy on the evolution of the early pyelonephritic scar. *Kidney International*, **20**, 733–742

Rolleston, G. L., Shannon, F. T. and Utley, W. L. F. (1970) Relationship of infantile vesico-ureteric reflux to renal damage. *British Medical Journal*, **1**, 460

White, R. H. R and Taylor, C. M. (1984) The nonoperative management of primary vesicoureteric reflux. In *Management of Vesicoureteric Reflux* (ed. J. H. Johnson), Williams and Wilkins, Baltimore, pp. 117–136

Haematuria

The investigations shown in the top row of Figure A2.1 are able to indicate diagnoses even when the history and clinical examination prove negative. Patients may present with discoloured urine or, when tested for other reasons, a urine sample of normal appearance may be positive on urinalysis. In either event microscopy will confirm haematuria and help separate it from haemoglobinuria or myoglobinuria. Microscopy may provide an immediate diagnosis as in the case of schistosomiasis or in the uncommon presentation by haematuria of a bacterial urinary tract infection. More usually, however, the value of microscopy is to indicate the site of bleeding, the presence of dysmorphic red cells or casts pointing to a renal parenchymal lesion.

If proteinuria coexists, the prospect of a parenchymal disorder is increased. Normal protein excretion, although making a rapidly progressive clinical course unlikely, does not completely exclude a potentially serious glomerular lesion such as Alport's syndrome. However, heavy proteinuria is associated with glomerular disease, especially proliferative lesions and focal segmental glomerulosclerosis. In such circumstances, measurement of complement components and antistreptococcal antibodies (antistreptolysin O titre (ASOT) and anti DNase-B) is indicated. A subnormal concentration of C_3 is seen in the acute phase of post streptococcal glomerulonephritis, but this typically recovers by 2 months. A persistent reduction is seen in membranoproliferative glomerulonephritis and sometimes in systemic lupus erythematosis. The glomerular filtration rate (GFR) should be monitored using the simple height/plasma creatinine formula and the results either tabulated or plotted graphically. Unless the diagnosis is clear from other clinical and laboratory findings, for example typical poststreptococcal nephritis, a renal biopsy should be performed.

Ultrasound examination combined with an abdominal X-ray is mandatory in all cases of haematuria and is good at identifying obstruction, calculus or tumour. In more advanced cases of glomerulonephritis or interstitial nephritis, the renal parenchyma

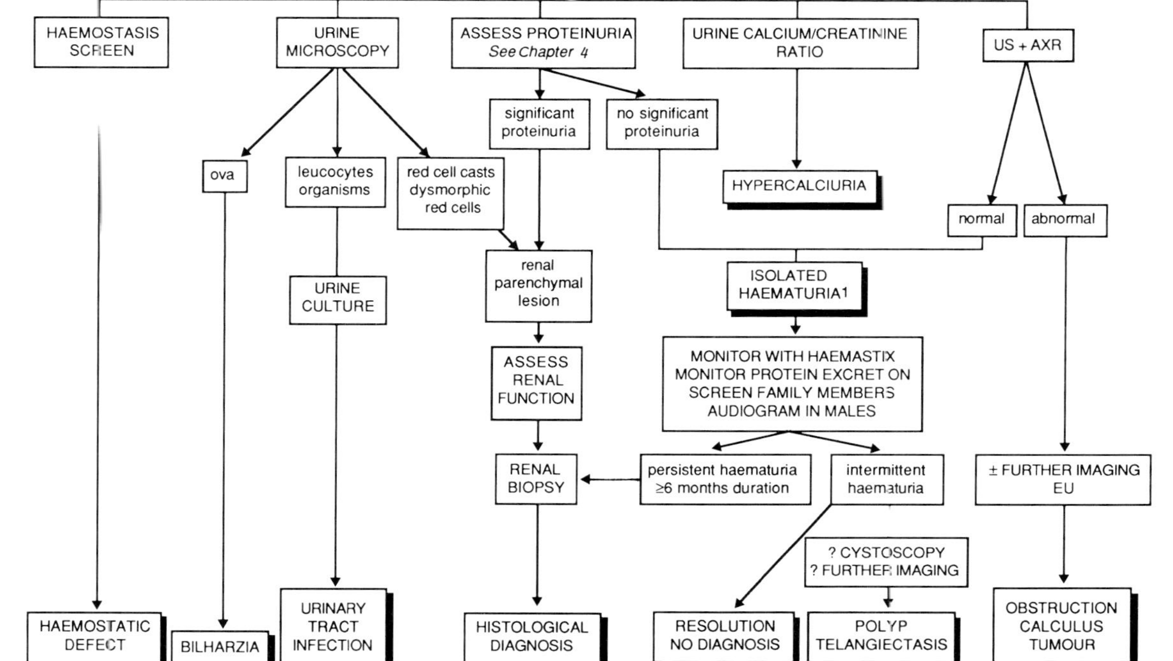

Figure A2.1 Algorithm for the investigation of haematuria. [1]In the absence of proteinuria a glomerular cause is likely to be either innocent or only slowly progressive

may show increased echogenicity. Unlike in adult medical practice, EU and cystoscopy are relegated to a lower place in Figure A2.1 as epithelial neoplasia is an extreme rarity in childhood.

Hypercalciuria has recently been recognized as an association of persistent microscopic haematuria in the absence of calculi (Stapleton *et al.*, 1984). The disorder is easy to identify (random urine calcium/creatinine ratio > 0.7 mmol mmol^{-1}), and with dietary calcium restriction and a high fluid intake the haematuria is said to resolve. Currently it is not certain that this is an exclusive association and other disorders may coexist.

A common problem is the investigation of a child with *isolated* microscopic haematuria, namely haematuria in the absence of proteinuria, functional impairment or gross structural abnormality. Isolated microscopic haematuria may be the residual abnormality in an individual who sustained subclinical acute nephritis. For this reason, in those patients without a family history it is helpful to monitor them at home with Haemastix at weekly intervals for a period of 6 months. If the haematuria resolves or is intermittent the prospect of finding a significant histological lesion is so remote that a biopsy is unnecessary. However, persistent haematuria of 6 months' duration demands investigation.

Broadly speaking, there are three main glomerular causes which need to be distinguished: IgA nephropathy, Alport's syndrome and benign familial nephritis. It is vital to obtain a complete family history and to test immediate family members for haematuria. Typical Alport's syndrome is an X-linked recessive disorder in which males get progressive neural deafness and end-stage renal failure by about 15–25 years of age. Females into middle life usually have microscopic haematuria only, and as this can be intermittent repeat screening of sisters and mothers should be undertaken. To confuse the issue there are families with a similar disorder of the glomerular basement membrane, who have normal hearing and probably a different pattern of inheritance; this has been called Alport variant. In benign familial haematuria, affected members show no renal decline over long periods of follow-up. Electron microscopy is essential for the diagnosis of the familial nephritides. Patients with Alport's syndrome exhibit thickening of the basement membrane with extensive replication of the lamina densa. In young children this may be preceded by an abnormally thin basement membrane. In some families with benign familial haematuria thin basement membranes only are found.

IgA nephropathy is a sporadic disease and a more common cause of isolated microscopic haematuria than are the familial conditions. The nephritis of Henoch–Schönlein purpura is histologically similar to IgA nephropathy and in this disease the usual renal manifestation is microscopic haematuria. One should always enquire specifically about a past illness of rash, joint and abdominal pain. Immuno-fluorescent biopsy staining is necessary to confirm these diagnoses.

Finally there will be a few patients who show no discernible histological abnormality.

Reference and further reading

Stapleton, F. B., Roy, S., Moe, H. N. and Jenkins, G. (1984) Hypercalcuria in children with hematuria. *New England Journal of Medicine*, **310**, 1345–1348
White, R. H. R. (1989) The investigation of haematuria. *Archives of Disease in Childhood*, **64**, 159–165

Proteinuria

An initial task is to distinguish between clinically significant proteinuria and that associated with fever, trauma, surgery or posture. The latter is excluded if an early morning urine protein/creatinine ratio is less then 20 mg mmol^{-1} (see Chapter 4).

Figure A3.1 shows that a height/plasma creatinine estimation of glomerular filtration rate (GFR), together with urine microscopy and ultrasound examination, readily leads towards diagnostic endpoints. The coexistence of haematuria suggests a renal parenchymal lesion, especially if the kidneys are of normal size and contour on ultrasound examination. Heavy proteinuria in these circumstances indicates a glomerular disorder whereas lesser amounts of proteinuria and a disproportionate reduction in GFR are more in keeping with a diffuse interstitial disease. In either event a renal biopsy will clarify the matter if other clinical clues have not already pinpointed the diagnosis.

Proteinuria is an inevitable consequence of chronic renal failure, irrespective of the cause. In conditions where renal mass is reduced, even though there is no active inflammatory process in the kidney, proteinuria may develop before there is any detectable decline in renal function. It is thought that proteinuria may be a marker of hyperperfusion in remaining glomeruli, and its sequential measurement is helpful in monitoring the clinical course of such patients (see Figure 4.1).

Ultrasonography (US) is a good screening test to identify reduced renal mass and some of the causative conditions. However, there may be difficulty in distinguishing between the coarse focal scarring of reflux nephropathy and renal dysplasia, for example. In such circumstances further clarification can be obtained by excretion urography and cystourethrography.

Ultrasound is valuable in identifying cystic renal disease. It should be noted that in adult-type polycystic kidney disease, cysts may not be discernible with this method until after 18 years of age, so that a negative result in childhood cannot be used to exclude the diagnosis.

Not all cases of renal vein thrombosis (RVT) can be identified by

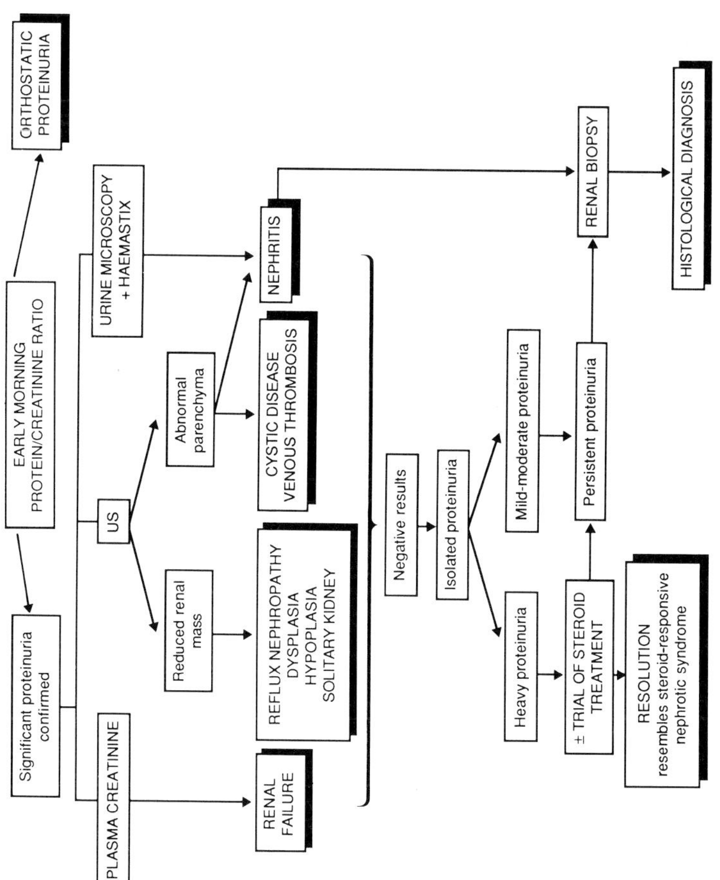

Figure A3.1 Algorithm for the investigation of proteinuria

US, but if thrombus extends into the renal veins or inferior vena cava this can often be seen.

Isolated heavy proteinuria

Heavy proteinuria without haematuria in an oedematous, normotensive child between 2 and 10 years of age is very likely to be due to minimal change nephrotic syndrome. Occasionally a child in this age-group presents with heavy proteinuria but no oedema. As long as renal function and US are normal, and there are no 'nephritic' features, it is justifiable to treat the child with prednisolone $2\,\mathrm{mg\,kg^{-1}\,day^{-1}}$ for a 4-week period to see if a remission of the proteinuria can be achieved, just as one would for a first episode of idiopathic nephrotic syndrome. If this abruptly arrests proteinuria, the prospects are that the child would have minimal change on a biopsy and therefore further invasive investigation is avoided. However, if proteinuria persists it is important to obtain a histological diagnosis.

Children presenting with heavy proteinuria in the first 6 months of life are rarely steroid sensitive and likely to have a congenital nephrotic syndrome. In these children a biopsy is mandatory. In teenagers, too, the prospect of finding steroid sensitivity is reduced as disorders such as focal segmental glomerular sclerosis, membranoproliferative glomerulonephritis and systemic lupus erythematosis take precedence. In these conditions the onset may be insidious and moderate proteinuria be found incidentally. Complement profile and antinuclear factor may help to indicate the diagnosis (see Chapter 13).

Hypertension

In the following indirect methods of blood pressure measurement, cuff size and position are important to avoid erroneous readings. For measurements in the upper arm the cuff should be the largest one which fits comfortably leaving sufficient room at the antecubital fossa to place the stethoscope over the brachial artery. The bladder should be centred over the artery and extend round more than half of the arm circumference. Small cuffs or bladders give artificially high readings and larger ones give low readings.

Auscultation is the traditional method of measurement. The cuff is rapidly inflated above systolic pressure and deflated at not more than 5 mmHg s^{-1}. The systolic pressure is that at which the first sounds are heard, the diastolic corresponds to the point of muffling (the fourth Korotkoff sound). Because auscultation is difficult in small children *ultrasound* devices using the Doppler principle are helpful. In these a transmitter/receiver is positioned directly over the brachial artery. Movement of blood in the artery is recognized and converted to an audible signal. As in auscultation the cuff is slowly deflated from above systolic pressure and the onset of pulse-like sounds is taken as the systolic reading. The change to a softer constant sound is regarded as the diastolic pressure.

The *flush method* is of value in infants when auscultation is difficult and other technologies are unavailable. The cuff is applied at the wrist or ankle. Before inflation the capillary bed of the hand or foot is compressed by applying an elastic bandage. The cuff is then inflated above systolic pressure and the compressive bandage released. On slowly deflating the cuff the point at which skin capillaries are reperfused is an estimate of the systolic blood pressure.

The newer automated technique of *plethysmography*, e.g. Dinamap (Critikon), is an extension of the old oscillometry technique. The material of the outer cuff and the hoses connecting it to the sensor are of non-compliant materials. Cuff inflation and deflation are controlled by a computer program. A pressure sensor detects volume displacement beneath the cuff from the pulsatile expansion of the artery. By plotting this against the cuff inflation pressure, systolic, diastolic and mean arterial pressures are computed and displayed. One of the advantages of this technique is that although cuff size remains important its position is less so. This method tends to overestimate actual arterial pressure in hypotensive babies weighing less than 1500 g (Diprose *et al.*, 1986).

Because blood pressure increases throughout childhood in relationship to age and body mass, measurements need to be interpreted using centile charts. Probably the most widely used are those produced by the Heart, Lung and Blood Institute Task Force (Blumenthal *et al.*, 1977). Because of the criticisms of Dillon (1988), we have here reproduced the centile charts of Andre *et al.* (1980) which have the advantage that they include standardization for height (Figure A4.1).

Depending on the centile chosen to define the upper limit of normal, some 1–3% of the population will have blood pressure recordings above this and will therefore be regarded as hypertensive. Where hypertension is mild it usually reflects essential hypertension. By contrast severe hypertension in childhood is almost invariably secondary. In infants of less than 1 year coarctation is the commonest cause, but beyond infancy renal disorders explain more than 80% of cases. Figure A4.2 illustrates a plan for investigating these cases.

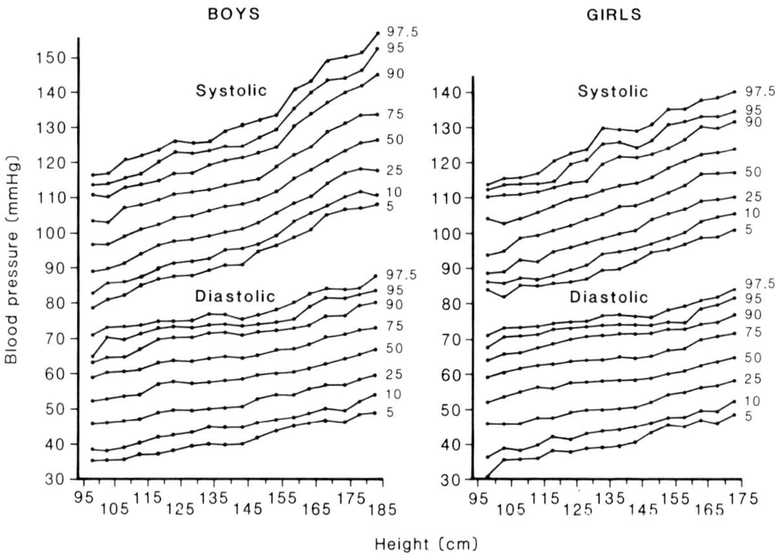

Figure A4.1 Centile charts for blood pressure in childhood

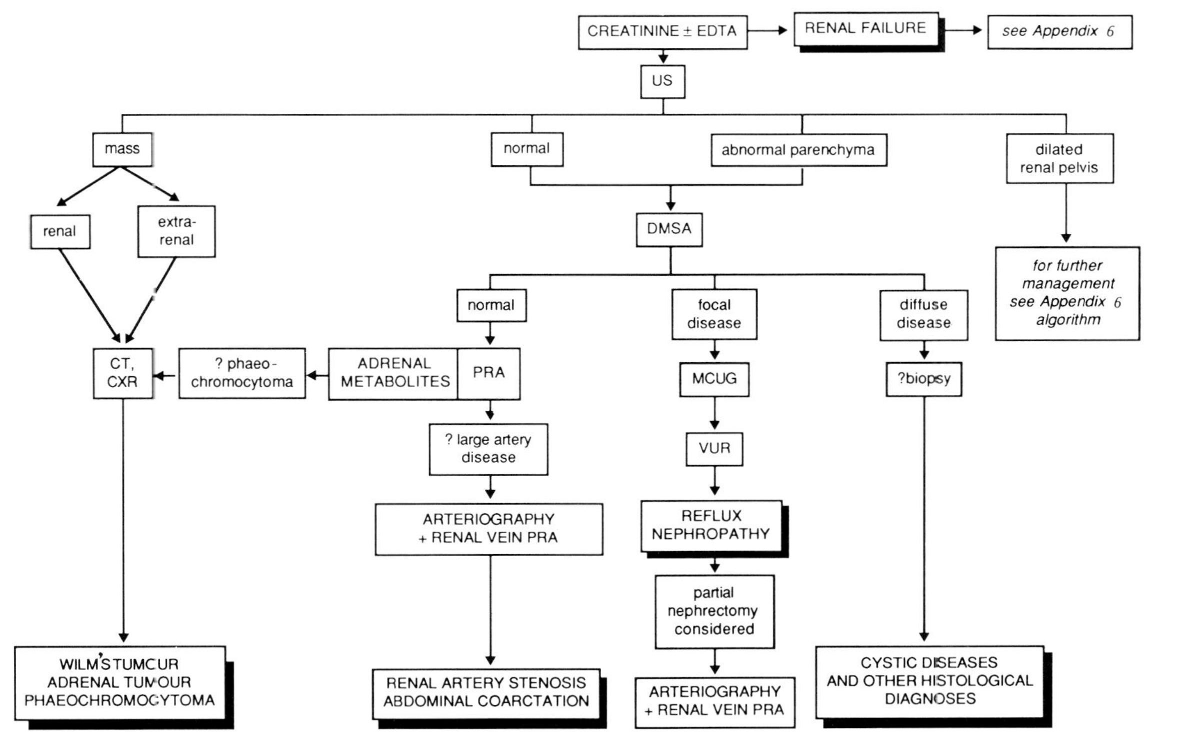

Figure A4.2 Algorithm for the investigation of hypertension

A height/creatinine estimation of glomerular filtration rate (GFR) and an ultrasound scan readily identify chronic renal failure, certain tumours, scarred and obstructed kidneys. Further imaging may be required as shown in Figure A4.2, and the following points should be noted.

Tc-DMSA scanning is the most sensitive indicator of a renal scar, whatever the aetiology (Dillon, Gordon and Shah, 1984) and photon-deficient areas correlate well with intrarenal vascular disease (Vivian *et al.*, 1982). Rosen and Treves (1983), in their evaluation of hypertensive paediatric and adolescent patients, found DMSA had a sensitivity of 92% and a specificity greater than 95%. When US and Tc-DMSA reveal two normal kidneys in the presence of raised peripheral venous plasma renin activity (PRA), main renal artery stenosis and abdominal coarctation remain to be excluded (Stringer *et al.*, 1984).

Evaluation of renal blood flow during the first phase of a *Tc-DTPA* renogram has been shown to be a poor technique for demonstrating main renal artery stenosis. However, in those patients with unilateral renal artery stenosis GFR may decrease markedly on the affected side during treatment with captopril (Wenting *et al.*, 1984). The finding of unilateral severe impairment of renal function during treatment with captopril should suggest this diagnosis.

The use of a rapid sequence of films during *excretion urography* (*the hypertensive urogram*) to monitor the arrival of contrast medium and thus diagnose main renal artery stenosis is now known to be inaccurate (Thornbury, Stanley and Fryback, 1982). Excretion urography should also not be used as an initial screening tool but rather to supplement US and/or a Tc-DMSA scan when the aetiology of a small kidney is still uncertain.

Micturating cystourethrography (MCUG) should be employed to determine if a small kidney or focal scar is due to vesico-ureteric reflux (VUR).

Arteriography and *renal vein sampling* should be undertaken in children who

1. have two normal kidneys as determined by US and Tc-DMSA and who have raised peripheral renin activity or catecholamines; or
2. are candidates for surgical relief of their hypertension; or
3. have an abnormal Tc-DMSA scan suggesting intrarenal renovascular disease (Gordon and Dillon, 1987).

Blood samples for PRA are taken from the inferior vena cava below the renal veins, both main renal veins and the segmental renal veins. A ratio between the main renal veins which exceeds 1.5:1 indicates renin-dependent hypertension (Gerdts *et al.*, 1979). Focal intrarenal abnormalities may be identified by elevated segmental renin vein ratios (SRVR). These are calculated by dividing the highest segmental vein PRA by lower segmental vein PRAs from the same kidney or from the contralateral kidney.

Arteriography is usually carried out immediately after renal vein sampling, with which it should be correlated. Injections of contrast medium into the abdominal aorta will show abdominal coarctation and stenosis at the origin of the renal artery. Selective renal artery injection will give improved definition of intrarenal arterial pathology, especially when combined with a magnification technique.

^{123}*I-meta-iodo-benzyl-guanidine* (MIBG) is a radiopharmaceutical which images cells which secrete catecholamines. It is a useful agent for the investigation of phaeochromocytoma and for imaging metastases from neuroblastoma.

Elevated peripheral venous *renin* measurements are found in patients with vascular or renal parenchymal disease and more rarely in renal tumours. To measure PRA the patient should be normally hydrated and supine for 2 hours prior to sampling. Low renin measurements are useful in excluding a renin-dependent state, and suppression by primary mineralocorticoid excess causes very low activity. If a test dose of captopril causes marked reduction in blood pressure this quickly gives a further indication of renin-mediated hypertension.

The excretion of the catecholamine derivative *vanillyl mandelic acid* (VMA) can be used as a marker for neuroblastoma and some phaeochromocytoma. However, not all phaeochromocytomas excrete VMA in excess and it is preferable to measure plasma *noradrenaline* which is constantly elevated.

Corticosteroid excess is a rare but important cause of hypertension. Where indicated urine *steroid analysis* or the direct measurement of plasma *aldosterone* and *cortisone* will distinguish Cushing's and Conn's syndromes and congenital adrenal hyperplasia (11-beta and 17-alpha-hydroxylase deficiency).

References

Andre, J. L., Deschamps, J. P. and Gueghen, R. (1980) La tension artérielle chez l'enfant et l'adolescent. Valeurs rapportées à l'âge et à la taille chez 17067 sujets. *Archives Françaises de Pédiatrie*, **37**, 477–482

Blumenthal, S., Epps, R. P., Heavenrich, R. *et al.* (1977) Report of the task force on blood pressure control in children. *Pediatrics*, **59**, (suppl.), 797–820

Dillon, M. J. (1988) Blood pressure. *Archives of Disease in Childhood*, **63**, 347–349

Dillon, M. J., Gordon, I. and Shah, V. (1984) ^{99m}Tc DMSA scanning and segmental renal vein renin estimation in children with renal scarring. In *Contributions to Nephrology* (ed. C. J. Hodson, J. Heptinstall and J. Winberg), Karger, Basel, pp. 20–27

Diprose, G. K., Evans, D. H., Archer, L. N. J. and Levene, M. I. (1986) Dinamap fails to detect hypotension in very low birthweight infants. *Archives of Disease in Childhood*, **61**, 771–773

Gerdts, K. G., Shah, V., Savage, J. M. and Dillon, M. J. (1979) Renal vein renin measurements in normotensive children. *Journal of Pediatrics*, **95**, 953–958

Gordon, I. and Dillon, M. J. (1987) Hypertension. In *Diagnostic Imaging in Paediatrics* (ed. I. Gordon), Chapman and Hall, London, pp. 163–174

Rosen, P. R. and Treves, S. (1983) The efficacy of Tc-99m DTPA and Tc-99m DMSA renography in the screening of paediatric patients for renal aetiologies in hypertension. *Journal of Nuclear Medicine*, **24**, 22

Stringer, D. A., de Bruyn, R., Dillon, M. J. and Gordon, I. (1984) Comparison of aortography, renal vein renin sampling, radionuclide scans and the IVU in the investigation of childhood renovascular hypertension. *British Journal of Radiology*, **57**, 111–121

Thornbury, J. R., Stanley, J. C. and Fryback, D. G. (1982) Hypertensive urogram: a nondiscriminatory test for renovascular hypertension. *American Journal of Roentgenology*, **138**, 43–49

Vivian, G., Stringer, D., de Bruyn, R. *et al.* (1982) 99mTc DMSA scans in renovascular hypertension in childhood. In *Proceedings of the Third World Congress of Nuclear Medicine and Biology* (Paris), Pergamon Press, Oxford, pp. 2663–2666

Wenting, G. J., Tan-Tjiong, H. L., Derkx, F. H. M. *et al.* (1984) Split renal function after captopril in unilateral renal artery stenosis. *British Medical Journal*, **288**, 886–890

Urolithiasis

In the investigation of a child with a urinary calculus the following questions need to be answered:

1. Is the calculus causing mechanical obstruction?
2. Is the urine infected?
3. What is the chemical nature of the stone and is there an underlying biochemical disorder?

The majority of calculi in the urinary tract contain sufficient calcium for their size and position to be identified easily on a plain abdominal X-ray. The exceptions are pure urate, cystine, and the rare xanthine and dihydroxyadenine stones. Together with a plain X-ray, an ultrasound scan is a good *screening* test for suspected calculus, being able to identify obstruction and major anatomical lesions. However, excretion urography is still the best method of exactly locating a calculus, radiolucent stones showing up as filling defects. Obstruction can usually be determined at the same time, but if there is doubt a ^{99m}Tc-DTPA renogram with frusemide diuresis may prove helpful.

Liaison with a paediatric urological surgeon should be sought in all cases. Wherever possible a urinary calculus should be recovered for chemical analysis. Patients need to have this explained to them so that if they pass the stone *per urethram* spontaneously they make an effort to retrieve it.

The majority of urinary calculi occurring in children in the United Kingdom are related to urinary tract stasis and infection, and contain either magnesium ammonium phosphate (struvite) or calcium phosphate (apatite). Urea-splitting organisms, particularly *Proteus* species, give rise to a high urinary pH which favours calcium deposition. Urinary debris may act as the nidus on which the triple phosphate calculus will grow. One-third of these patients have associated urological abnormalities and preschool aged boys are most often affected (Ghazali *et al.*, 1973). Infection must be rigorously controlled, especially where obstruction coexists, as together these can cause rapid renal parenchymal destruction.

In the United Kingdom the prospect of identifying a primary biochemical disorder is less than 10%, but in other countries, such as the USA where infection-related stones are less common, the proportion with a metabolic disorder is greater. If a primary disease is suggested by the stone analysis, confirmation of the underlying disorder should be undertaken. If the calculus cannot be recovered or has been lost it is worth screening the patient with the following investigations.

1. *Plasma creatinine* to estimate GFR from the child's height.
2. *Plasma bicarbonate and urine pH* to identify renal tubular acidosis. Nephrocalcinosis is a complication of inadequately treated renal tubular acidosis.
3. *Plasma calcium, phosphorus and alkaline phosphatase*: unlike adult practice, hypercalcaemic states, particularly primary hyperparathyroidism, are rare. However Williams' syndrome and vitamin D intoxication should be considered.
4. *Urine calcium/creatinine ratio*: a consistent ratio of >0.7 mmol mmol^{-1} indicates hypercalciuria.
5. Twenty-four hour urine collection for *oxalate, uric acid and cystine*. Unfortunately there are as yet no usable normal data on ratios of these products to urinary creatinine and therefore complete and exactly timed urine saves are needed. Always confirm the reference range with the laboratory performing the test; the following upper limits are for outline guidance only:

Oxalate	0.33 mmol per 1.73 m^2 per 24 h
Uric acid	5 mmol per 1.73 m^2 per 24 h
Cystine	0.42 mmol per 1.73 m^2 per 24 h.

Reference and further reading

Chambers, T. L. (1986) Renal stones and nephrocalcinosis. In *Clinical Paediatric Nephrology* (ed. R. J. Postlethwaite), Wright, Bristol, pp. 394–403
Ghazali, S., Barratt, T. M. and Williams, D. I. (1973) Childhood urolithiasis in Britain. *Archives of Disease in Childhood*, **48**, 291–295
Marshall, V. R. and Ryall, R. L. (1981) Investigation of urinary calculi. *British Journal of Hospital Medicine*, **26**, 389–392

Renal failure

Renal failure may be acute, acute on chronic or chronic, and aetiologically the causes may be considered under three main headings, namely pre-renal (i.e. hypoperfusion), renal (i.e. intrinsic) and postrenal (obstructive uropathy). There are no pre-renal causes of chronic renal failure and as this group does not present a diagnostic problem they will be excluded from this discussion. In evaluating the child who presents in renal failure a number of questions need to be answered.

1. Is this acute, acute-on-chronic or chronic renal failure?
Signs indicative of chronicity include (in order of chronicity) growth retardation, renal osteodystrophy and anaemia, and their presence will indicate a chronic or acute-on-chronic process. Radiographs of the hand and wrist and knee should be examined for evidence of metabolic bone disease (see Chapter 8) and for determination of bone age. Urine culture and microscopy are mandatory to exclude a urinary tract infection which may explain an acute deterioration of renal function in a child with pre-existent renal impairment.

2. How many kidneys are present and are they large, small or of normal size?
This question is answered by US, which is the ideal imaging tool in renal failure because of its non-dependence on renal function. It is important to assess overall renal mass because if two kidneys are present then there must be bilateral renal disease for renal failure to have occurred. Kidneys which are of normal or increased size will need to be biopsied unless the patient already has a primary diagnosis such as acute lymphoblastic leukaemia.

3. What is the renal parenchyma like?
Increased renal echogenicity and/or abnormal corticomedullary differentiation on US imply a renal cause for the renal failure. In the presence of bilateral echogenic kidneys, if MCUG does not demonstrate vesico-ureteric reflux (VUR) then the most likely diagnosis is

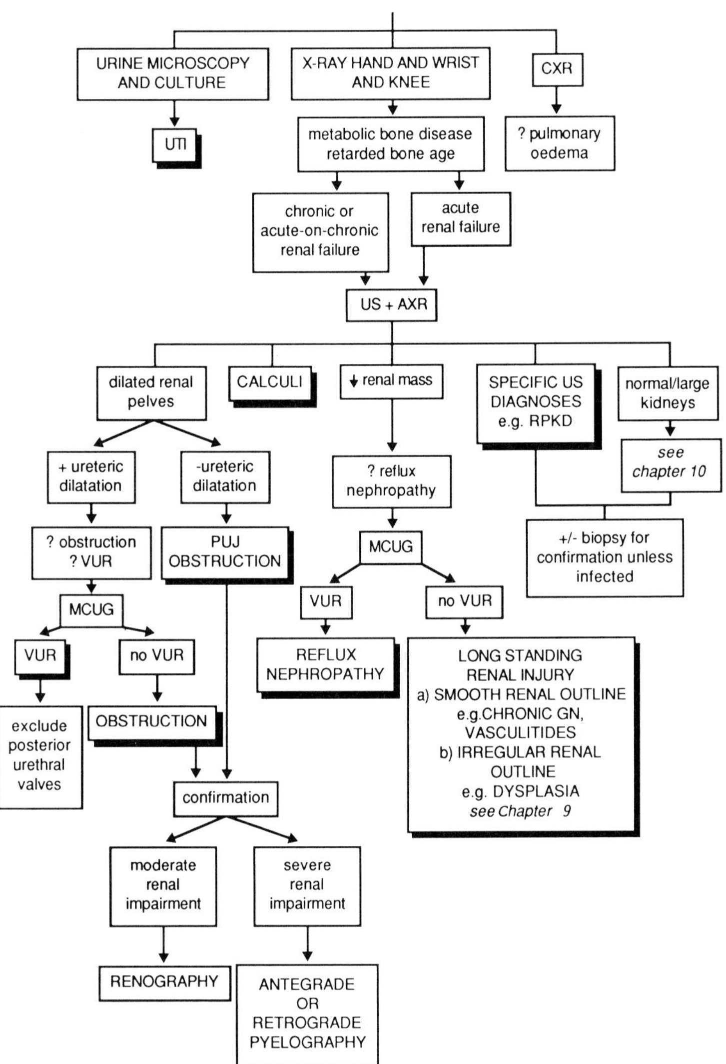

Figure A6.1 Algorithm for the investigation of renal failure

renal dysplasia. Causes of bilaterally large smooth kidneys and scarred kidneys are given in Chapter 9.

4. Are the collecting systems dilated?
This is also answered by US (Denton, Cochlin and Evans, 1984). Postrenal causes of renal failure are the most important to diagnose

because this is the group most amenable to treatment. Differentiation between obstructive nephropathy and reflux nephropathy will depend on the level of dilatation and, if the ureters are dilated, on the results of other imaging tests such as MCUG and retrograde or antegrade pyeloureterography. It must be remembered that uncommonly obstructive uropathy may occur without dilatation (Lyons, Matthews and Evans, 1988). This situation has been reported following surgery to the urinary tract, in association with retroperitoneal fibrosis, pelvic and retroperitoneal malignancies and in obstruction due to ureteric calculi.

5. Are there calculi or renal calcifications?
Radio-opaque calculi will be identified on the plain abdominal radiograph and confirmed by US.

6. Is there any spinal abnormality to suggest the presence of a neuropathic bladder?

It should be noted that Tc-DTPA and Tc-DMSA scans are of limited value in severe renal failure because they are dependent on functioning renal tissue.

Figure A6.1 illustrates a suggested algorithm for the investigation of renal failure.

References

Denton, T., Cochlin, D. L. and Evans, C. (1984) The value of ultrasound in previously undiagnosed renal failure. *British Journal of Radiology,* **57,** 673–675

Lyons, K., Matthews, P. and Evans, C. (1988) Obstructive uropathy without dilatation: a potential diagnostic pitfall. *British Medical Journal,* **296,** 1517–1518

Neonatal renal mass

In the newborn period the majority of abdominal masses represent benign disorders of development, and 55% are of renal origin (Griscom, 1965). During this period when impaired renal function limits the usefulness of excretion urography (EU), real-time ultrasonography (US), which provides structural information, and radionuclide imaging for functional assessment have revolutionized the investigation of these infants. A recent review is provided by Merten and Kirks (1985). The most common causes of a neonatal renal mass(es) are now listed.

Hydronephrosis (25%)

The most common cause is pelvi-ureteric junction (PUJ) obstruction (22%) followed by posterior urethral valves (18%), ureterovesical junction obstruction and vesico-ureteric reflux (Lebowitz and Griscom, 1977). In our experience the majority are now picked up by antenatal US. Those who present postnatally may have an asymptomatic loin mass or develop a complicating urinary tract infection.

Multicystic dysplastic kidney (15%)

Ultrasonography will show multiple anechoic cysts of similar or variable size, which do not communicate with each other, and radionuclide imaging shows no activity within the affected kidney (Figure A7.1(b)). One-third of patients have a contralateral renal abnormality, PUJ obstruction being the most common.

Recessive polycystic kidney disease (RPKD)

Ultrasonography demonstrates bilateral nephromegaly with a bright echonephrogram (see Figure 10.19). This increased echogenicity is due to the microcysts increasing the number of interfaces which can reflect back the sound. In addition, it may be possible to discern small macrocysts.

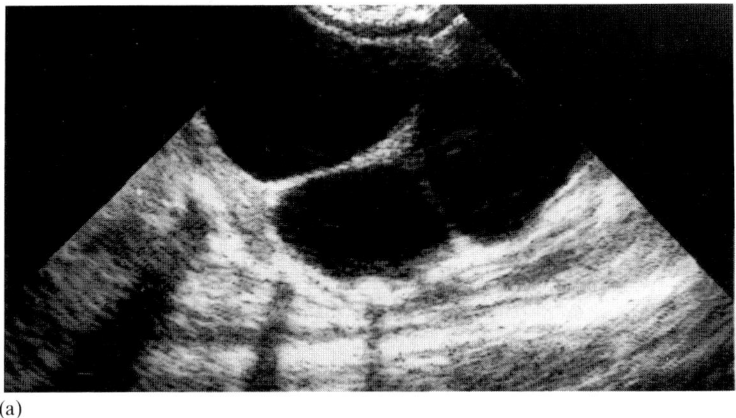

(a)

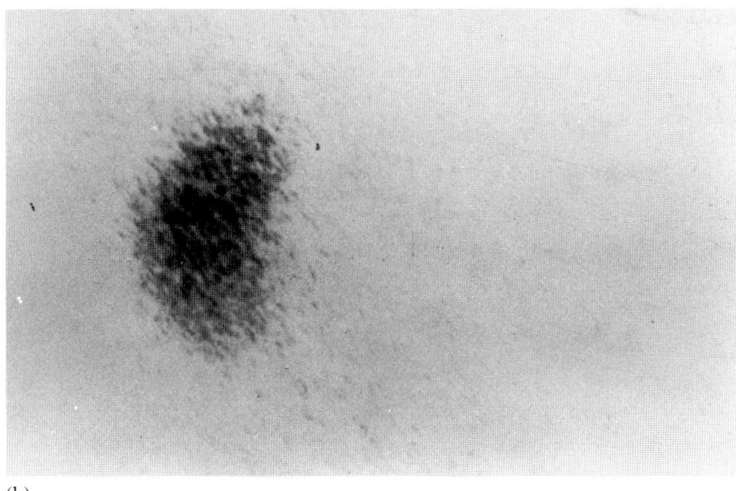

(b)

Figure A7.1 A multicystic kidney. (a) The longitudinal US scan shows a number of discrete, non-communicating cysts with a very thin rim of renal parenchyma. (b) Tc-DMSA scintigraphy shows no renal activity on that side.

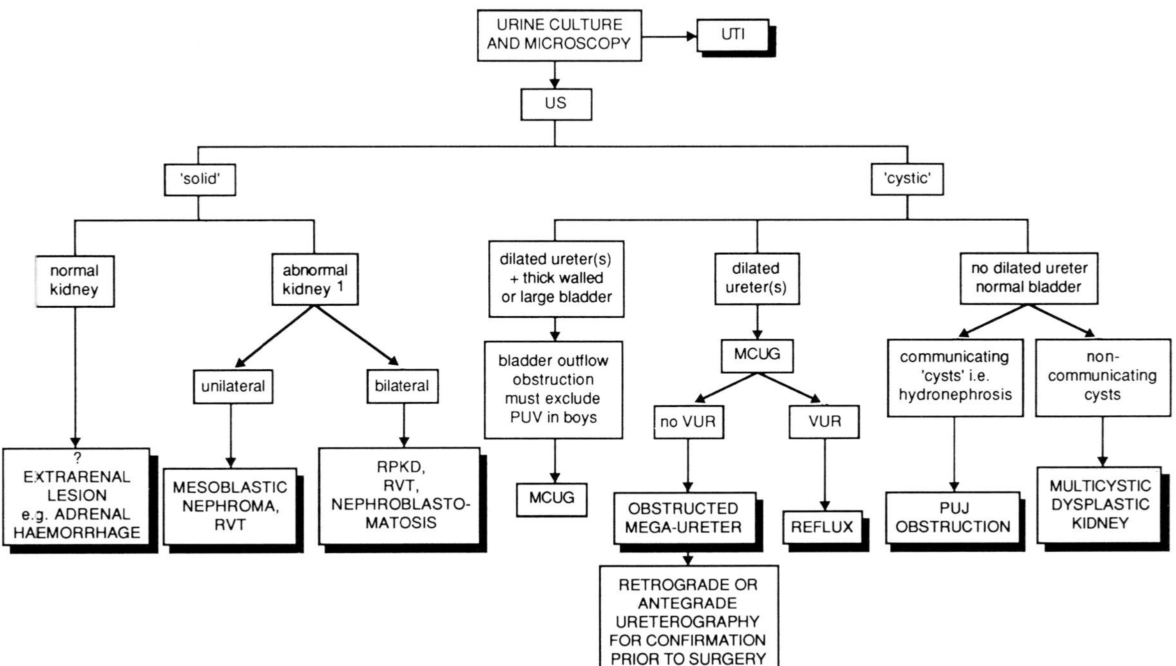

Figure A7.2 Algorithm for the investigation of neonatal renal mass. [1]See Table 10.2

Renal vein thrombosis (RVT)

This may complicate dehydration, shock, septicaemia, cyanotic congenital heart disease or maternal diabetes mellitus. Ultrasonography reveals uni- or bilateral renal enlargement with a mixed echo pattern. Areas of high echogenicity represent haemorrhage and areas of low echogenicity are due to oedema. Corticomedullary differentiation is destroyed (see Figure 10.11).

Mesoblastic nephroma

This is a benign renal neoplasm which accounts for nearly all neonatal renal tumours rather than Wilms' tumour.

A simple algorithm is illustrated in Figure A7.2, the aims of imaging being to confirm the renal origin of the mass and to determine whether it is solid or cystic. Further tabulation of the different renal parenchymal abnormalities found on US is given in Table 10.2. Renal function is best assessed with Tc-DTPA renography.

References

Griscom, N. T. (1965) The roentgenology of neonatal abdominal masses. *American Journal of Roentgenology*, **93**, 447–463

Lebowitz, R. L. and Griscom, N. T. (1977) Neonatal hydronephrosis: 146 cases. *Radiologic Clinics of North America*, **15**, 49–59

Merten, D. F. and Kirks, D. R. (1985) Diagnostic imaging of paediatric abdominal masses. *Pediatric Clinics of North America*, **32**, 1397–1425

Index